Reflux Laryngitis and Related Disorders

Fourth Edition

Reflux Laryngitis and Related Disorders

Fourth Edition

Robert T. Sataloff, MD, DMA, FACS

Philip O. Katz, MD

Mary J. Hawkshaw, BSN, RN, CORLN

Dahlia M. Sataloff, MD, FACS

Plural Publishing Inc.
San Diego
Oxford
Melbourne

PLURAL PUBLISHING INC.

5521 Ruffin Road
San Diego, CA 92123

e-mail: info@pluralpublishing.com
Web site: http://www.pluralpublishing.com

Typeset in 10/12 Palatino by Flanagan's Publishing Services, Inc.
Printed in the United States of America by McNaughton & Gunn, Inc.

NOTICE TO THE READER

Care has been taken to confirm the accuracy of the indications, procedures, drug dosages, and diagnosis and remediation protocols presented in this book and to ensure that they conform to the practices of the general medical and health services communities. However, the authors, editors, and publisher are not responsible for errors or omissions or for any consequences from application of the information in this book and make no warranty, expressed or implied, with respect to the currency, completeness, or accuracy of the contents of the publication. The diagnostic and remediation protocols and the medications described do not necessarily have specific approval by the Food and Drug administration for use in the disorders and/or diseases and dosages for which they are recommended. Application of this information in a particular situation remains the professional responsibility of the practitioner. Because standards of practice and usage change, it is the responsibility of the practitioner to keep abreast of revised recommendations, dosages, and procedures.

Library of Congress Cataloging-in-Publication Data

Sataloff, Robert Thayer, author.
Reflux laryngitis and related disorders / Robert T. Sataloff, Philip Katz, Mary J. Hawkshaw, Dahlia Sataloff, authors. -- Fourth edition.
p. ; cm.
Includes bibliographical references and index.
ISBN-13: 978-1-59756-538-7 (alk. paper)
ISBN-10: 1-59756-538-5 (alk. paper)
I. Katz, Philip O., 1953- author. II. Hawkshaw, Mary, author. III. Sataloff, Dahlia, author. IV. Title.
[DNLM: 1. Laryngitis--diagnosis. 2. Laryngitis--etiology. 3. Laryngopharyngeal Reflux--complications. 4. Laryngopharyngeal Reflux--therapy. WY 510]
RF510
616.2'2--dc23

2013011269

Contents

Preface

Reflux laryngitis is an extremely common condition that is often overlooked. Because patients with reflux laryngitis and other symptoms and signs of laryngopharyngeal reflux often do not experience heartburn, many patients and their physicians do not recognize that these symptoms are being caused by gastroesophageal reflux disease. Because reflux is so frequently responsible for hoarseness, halitosis, symptoms of "postnasal drip," recurrent sore throat, chronic cough, reactive airway symptoms, and other common maladies, it is useful for all health care providers to be familiar with reflux laryngitis and related disorders. Such familiarity is especially important because ongoing, longstanding reflux can increase the risk for Barett's esophagus, esophageal adenocarcinoma, and cancer of the larynx.

This book provides a practical overview of reflux laryngitis and other manifestations of laryngopharyngeal reflux. It is designed for use by otolaryngologists, primary care physicians, internists, gastroenterologists, general surgeons, speech-language pathologists, voice teachers, and patients. Since the first edition of this book was written, there has been a great deal of interest in laryngopharyngeal reflux. Research has revealed new information; diagnostic and treatment paradigms have changed; and new medical and surgical therapies have been developed. The fourth edition of this book highlights these new developments and cites many articles that were not referenced in the third edition. We hope that readers will find this updated information interesting and valuable in their efforts to provide patients with optimal management for laryngopharyngeal reflux.

Chapter 1 introduces laryngopharyngeal reflux as a multisystem disorder and defines its importance in otolaryngologic and pulmonary conditions. Chapter 2 summarizes the complex structure and function of the human voice, laying the scientific groundwork necessary to understand the ways in which reflux can impair voice use. Chapter 3 defines esophageal structures and function, providing a comprehensive review of the mechanisms of swallowing and a concise discussion of the physiology of the lower esophageal sphincter. Chapter 4 is a new addition to this book and discusses new concepts in esophageal anatomy and the antireflux barrier. Chapter 5 reviews the symptoms associated with not only typical gastroesophageal reflux disease but also atypical (extraesophageal) reflux, including laryngopharyngeal reflux complaints and other symptoms such as chest pain. This chapter also reviews complications of reflux such as Barrett's esophagus and includes new information on diagnostic technology. Chapter 6 provides a comprehensive discussion of laryngopharyngeal reflux and the symptoms and signs associated with peptic mucositis of the larynx and related structures. This chapter also updates much of the literature on laryngopharyngeal reflux and stresses some particularly important reflux-related conditions such as laryngeal granuloma. Chapter 7 reviews the diagnostic tests available for patients with suspected reflux and the uses, strengths, and shortcomings of each procedure. It includes an extensive review of recent publications on this topic. Chapter 8 reviews the latest concepts in and literature on medical and behavioral management of reflux disease. Chapter 9 describes surgery for reflux, including an in-depth explanation of laparoscopic antireflux surgery illustrated by surgeon-medical illustrator John Potochny, MD, as well as a discussion of endoscopic approaches to reflux management.

In an effort to make this book useful for both health care providers and reflux sufferers, we have tried to keep this text clear and concise. We hope that this book will increase awareness of laryngopharyngeal reflux and its importance in clinical practice as well as provide practitioners with a convenient synopsis of the latest advances in diagnosis and treatment of laryngopharyngeal reflux.

Robert T. Sataloff, MD, DMA, FACS
Philip O. Katz, MD
Mary J. Hawkshaw, BSN, RN, CORLN
Dahlia M. Sataloff, MD, FACS

About the Authors

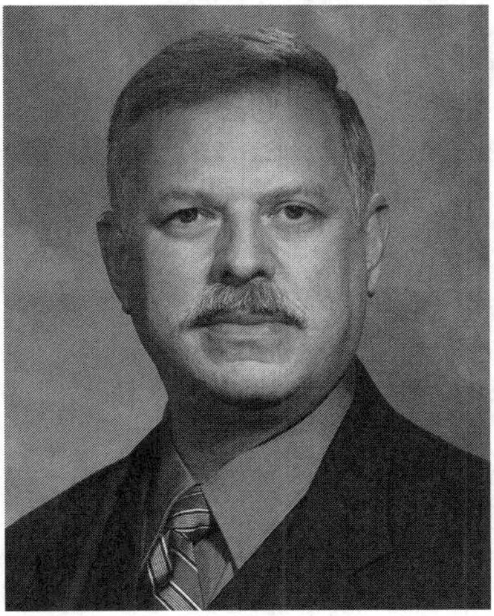

Robert Thayer Sataloff, MD, DMA, FACS

Robert T. Sataloff, MD, DMA, FACS, is professor and chairman of the Department of Otolaryngology—Head and Neck Surgery and senior associate dean for Clinical Academic Specialties, Drexel University College of Medicine. He is also adjunct professor in the Department of Otolaryngology—Head and Neck Surgery at Thomas Jefferson University, the University of Pennsylvania, and Temple University, and is on the faculty of the Academy of Vocal Arts. Dr. Sataloff is also a professional singer and singing teacher, and he served as conductor of the Thomas Jefferson University Choir for nearly 4 decades. He holds an undergraduate degree from Haverford College in music theory and composition, graduated from Jefferson Medical College, Thomas Jefferson University, received a doctor of musical arts in voice performance from Combs College of Music, and he completed his residency in otolaryngology—head and neck surgery and a fellowship in otology, neurotology and skull base surgery at the University of Michigan. Dr. Sataloff is chairman of the boards of directors of the Voice Foundation and of the American Institute for Voice and Ear Research. He has also served as chairman of the board of governors of Graduate Hospital; as president of the American Laryngological Association, the International Association of Phonosurgery and the Pennsylvania Academy of Otolaryngology–Head and Neck Surgery; and in numerous other leadership positions.

Dr. Sataloff is editor-in-chief of the *Journal of Voice*, editor-in-chief of *Ear, Nose and Throat Journal*, editor-in-chief of the *Journal of Case Reports in Medicine*, associate editor of the *Journal of Singing*, and on the editorial boards of numerous otolaryngology journals. He has written more than 1,000 publications, including 45 books. His medical practice is limited to care of the professional voice and to otology/neurotology/skull base surgery.

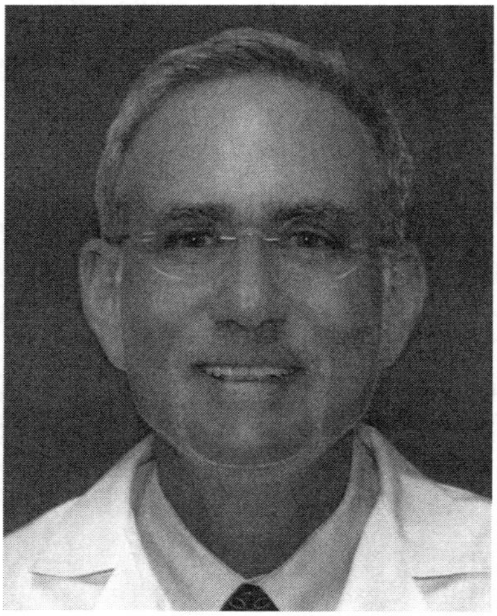

Philip O. Katz, MD

Philip O. Katz, MD, is a clinical professor of medicine at Jefferson Medical College and chairman of the Division of Gastroenterology at Einstein Medical Center in Philadelphia, Pennsylvania. He is also associate program director of the Department of Medicine at Albert Einstein Medical Center.

Dr. Katz received his medical degree from the Bowman Gray School of Medicine at Wake Forest University in Winston-Salem, North Carolina. He served his residency and chief residency in internal medicine, followed by a fellowship in gastroenterology at the Bowman Gray School of Medicine. He completed a faculty development fellowship at Johns Hopkins University in Baltimore, Maryland. He is board certified in internal medicine and gastroenterology.

Dr. Katz is the past president of the American College of Gastroenterology (2009–2010) and is a member of the American Gastroenterological Association and the American Society for Gastrointestinal Endoscopy.

A recognized national authority on esophageal disease, Dr. Katz's research interests focus on all aspects of gastroesophageal reflux disease, including nocturnal recovery of gastric acid secretion during proton-pump inhibitor therapy and esophageal pain perception. Dr. Katz is a practicing clinician with active teaching and editorial positions. In addition to lecturing on many gastroenterology-related topics, Dr. Katz is an editorial reviewer for *Annals of Internal Medicine, American Journal of Gastroenterology, Gastroenterology,* and *Digestive Diseases and Sciences.* He has contributed to the publication of more than 160 peer-reviewed papers, as well as numerous abstracts, book chapters, and monographs.

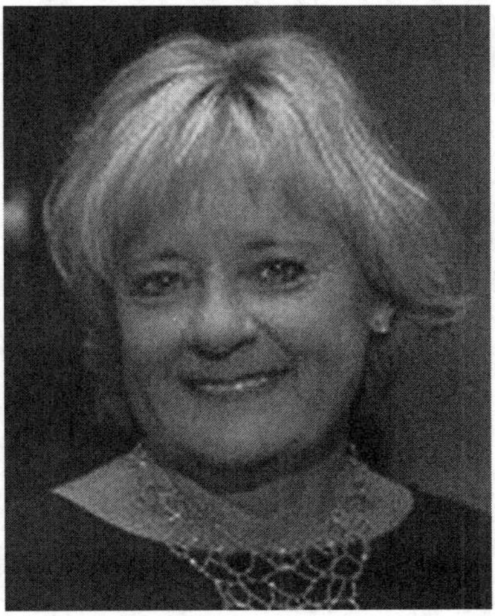

Mary J. Hawkshaw, BSN, RN, CORLN

Mary J. Hawkshaw, BSN, RN, CORLN, is a research associate professor in the Department of Otolaryngology—Head and Neck Surgery at Drexel University College of Medicine. She has been in association with Dr. Robert Sataloff, Philadelphia Ear, Nose and Throat Associates, and the American Institute for Voice and Ear Research (AIVER) since 1986. She has served as secretary and treasurer of AIVER since 1988 and was named executive director of AIVER in January 2000. She has served on the board of directors of the Voice Foundation since 1990. Ms. Hawkshaw graduated from Shadyside Hospital School of Nursing in Pittsburgh, Pennsylvania and received a bachelor of science degree in nursing from Thomas Jefferson University in Philadelphia. In collaboration with Dr. Sataloff, she has co-authored more than 65 book chapters, 160 articles, and 7 textbooks. She is on the editorial boards of the *Journal of Voice* and the *Ear, Nose, and Throat Journal.* She has been an active member of the Society of Otolaryngologic Head and Neck Nurses since 1998. She is recognized nationally and internationally for her extensive contributions to care of the professional voice.

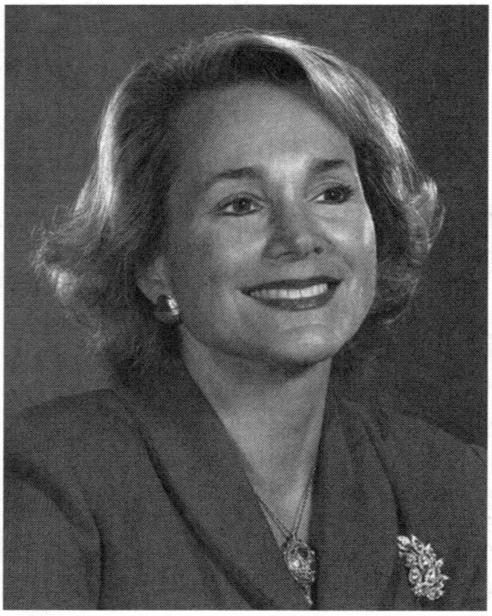

Dahlia M. Sataloff, MD, FACS

Dahlia M. Sataloff, MD, FACS, is a clinical professor in the Department of Surgery at the University of Pennsylvania's Perelman School of Medicine, and chair of the Department of Surgery and director of the Integrated Breast Center at Pennsylvania Hospital. Dr. Sataloff is an honors graduate from the University of Michigan Medical School and completed her residency in surgery at Pennsylvania Hospital. Board-certified in general surgery and a fellow of the American College of Surgeons, she is also a member of many professional societies including the American Society of Clinical Oncology, Society of Surgical Oncology, and the American Society of Breast Surgeons, among others. She serves as an editorial reviewer for the *Archives of Surgery* and is a member of the Eastern Cooperative Oncology Group.

Dr. Sataloff's practice is now devoted exclusively to breast surgery and management of benign and malignant breast diseases. She has lectured extensively on breast cancer detection as well as treatment and management, and is the author of more than 30 scientific papers and 4 books. Prior to limiting her practice to breast surgery, Dr. Sataloff was involved extensively in treatment of reflux disease and was one of the first surgeons to perform laparoscopic fundoplication. Dr. Sataloff is the recipient of many awards and has been recognized as one of *Philadelphia Magazine's* "Top Docs" for the treatment of breast disease as well as Castle Connolly's America's Top Doctors for Cancer.

Contributors

Mary J. Hawkshaw, BSN, RN, CORLN
Research Associate Professor
Department of Otolaryngology—Head and Neck Surgery
Drexel University College of Medicine
Otolaryngologic Nurse Clinician
Philadelphia Ear, Nose and Throat Associates
Executive Director
American Institute for Voice and Ear Research
Board of Directors
The Voice Foundation
Philadelphia, PA

Philip O. Katz, MD
Clinical Professor of Medicine
Jefferson Medical College
Chairman of Gastroenterology
Associate Program Director
Department of Medicine
Einstein Medical Center
Philadelphia, PA

Kian Makipour
Temple University
Ambler, PA
Chapter 4

Pathikonda Murali
Temple University
Ambler, PA
Chapter 4

Larry Miller, MD
Professor of Medicine
Chief of Gastroenterology
Hofstra University Medical School
Professor of Medicine
The Feinstein Research Institute
Chief of Gastroenterology
Digestive Disease Institute of the Division of Gastroenterology, Hepatology, and Nutrition
North Shore Long Island Jewish Medical Center
New Hyde Park, NY
Chapter 4

Dahlia Sataloff, MD, FACS
Clinical Professor and Vice Chair
Department of Surgery
University of Pennsylvania's Perelman School of Medicine
Chair
Department of Surgery
Director
Integrated Breast Center
Pennsylvania Hospital
Philadelphia, PA

Robert T. Sataloff, MD, DMA, FACS
Professor and Chairman
Senior Associate Dean for Clinical Academic Specialties
Department of Otolaryngology—Head and Neck Surgery
Drexel University College of Medicine
Chairman
The Voice Foundation
Chairman
American Institute for Voice and Ear Research
Philadelphia, PA

Anil Vegesna, MD
Hofstra University Medical School
The Feinstein Research Institute
Digestive Disease Institute of the Division of Gastroenterology, Hepatology, and Nutrition
North Shore Long Island Jewish Medical Center
New Hyde Park, NY
Chapter 4

To our families.

1

Introduction

Laryngopharyngeal reflux (LPR) is gastroesophageal reflux disease (GERD) that affects the pharynx and larynx. Reflux laryngitis (RL) is only one component of LPR. LPR and RL are diagnoses that remain subjects for debate because their symptomatology and clinical manifestations are not the same as those of GERD. In fact, discussion of RL and LPR in the otolaryngology literature prior to the 1970s and 1980s is almost nonexistent. During those decades, however, several reports of LPR and GERD were published.[1–15] Usually, when RL is present, symptoms and signs of more generalized LPR are also present, although they are commonly missed if not elicited by specific questions during the medical history and by meticulous physical examination.

Occult chronic gastroesophageal reflux is an etiologic factor in a high percentage of patients of all ages with laryngologic (ie, voice) complaints. Wiener et al[16] reported in 1989 that 78% of patients in a series of 32 patients had LPR documented on dual-probe pH monitoring studies. It has also been found to be a particularly common problem in professional voice users and singers. In 1991, Sataloff et al[17] reported RL in 265 of 583 consecutive professional voice users (45%), including singers and others who sought medical care during a 12-month period. However, RL was often diagnosed incidentally and was not always responsible for the patient's primary voice complaint. The incidence of RL may be lower in patients with other vocations, but it is of interest that Koufman et al[18] found gastroesophageal reflux in 78% of patients with hoarseness and in about 50% of all patients with voice complaints. Other reports have been published on the pathogenesis of voice disorders and otolaryngologic manifestations of LPR and its prevalence.[19–32] Nevertheless, the prevalence of LPR in all patients who seek evaluation for voice complaints remains unknown. Additional epidemiologic studies are needed to help clarify the clinical importance of this entity.

LPR involves multiple anatomic sites, including the sphincter between the stomach and the distal esophagus; the entire length of the esophagus; the upper esophageal sphincter; the structures of the larynx, pharynx, and oral cavity; and the trachea and lungs. Consequently, it should be evident that LPR is managed best using a multidisciplinary team approach. The optimal team includes at least a laryngologist, an internist or primary care physician, and a gastroenterologist, together with supporting laboratory personnel, a speech-language pathologist, and a pulmonologist. For voice professionals, a singing voice specialist and an acting voice specialist should be included.[33] The availability of a knowledgeable psychologist and a nutritionist is highly desirable as well.[33,34] Although it is possible for one physician to manage most or all aspects of LPR, this approach does not provide comprehensive state-of-the-art care.

Laryngeal involvement by GERD commonly results in dysphonia for which patients attempt to compensate through hyperfunctional voice use patterns (muscular tension dysphonia). The collaboration of a speech-language pathologist and other voice team members is invaluable in eliminating compensatory behaviors and optimizing phonatory technique. Although laryngologists can certainly purchase 24-hour pH monitoring equipment and may even perform manometry, they do not generally do so with the same level of expertise as does a gastroenterologist, whose entire career may be devoted to disorders of the esophagus. Just as certain laryngologists subspecialize in voice care, some gastroenterologists subspecialize in the management of reflux. This group of professionals and their ancillary staff may be best equipped to diagnose gastroesophageal reflux and its consequences.

LPR is almost always associated with some degree of aspiration, which may be clinically insignificant or may cause chronic cough, reactive airway disease, difficulties controlling asthma, pneumonia, or bronchiectasis. A knowledgeable pulmonologist is essential in recognizing and treating these conditions.

Several issues are of special concern in the management of otolaryngologic patients with RL, especially professional voice users. First, many of these patients are young and will require prolonged or lifetime use of high doses of histamine type 2 receptor antagonists or proton-pump inhibitors. Although these agents are quite safe, the ultimate long-term effects of such medications over time are unknown. Moreover, the drugs are expensive; the cost may be burdensome, and financial strain often leads to poor compliance. Second, medications do not eliminate or cure reflux. They simply neutralize the refluxate, thereby controlling the symptoms effectively in many patients. However, some patients may continue to aspirate pH-neutral fluid, bile salts, and other substances not appropriate for entry into the pharynx, larynx, and lungs. In professional singers and other high-performance voice users, this problem may continue to be symptomatic (as throat clearing, excess phlegm, or cough), even when acidity is controlled well, although no one has demonstrated that deacidified gastric acid actually causes mucosal injury.

As stated, medications do not cure reflux; however, surgery may actually eliminate reflux. Conveniently, surgical therapy for GERD has improved dramatically with the advent of laparoscopic Nissen fundoplication and endoscopic antireflux procedures that offer alternatives to chronic medical management. An increasing percentage of patients are being referred for surgical treatment.

It is essential for the otolaryngologist to be familiar with the relevant anatomy, physiology, and pathology and with diagnosis and treatment options for LPR and GERD in general. Although much of this knowledge is outside traditional otolaryngology training, familiarity with the latest concepts and techniques in the management of GERD and RL in voice patients helps the otolaryngologist assemble an appropriate team and ensure optimal patient care.

REFERENCES

1. Olson NR. The problem of gastroesophageal reflux. *Otolaryngol Clin North Am.* 1986;19:119–133.
2. Menon AP, Schefft GL, Thach BT. Apnea associated with regurgitation in infants. *J Pediatr.* 1985;106:625–629.
3. Little FB, Koufman JA, Kohut RI, Marshall RB. Effect of gastric acid on the pathogenesis of subglottic stenosis. *Ann Otol Rhinol Laryngol.* 1985;94:516–519.
4. Kambic V, Radsel Z. Acid posterior laryngitis. Aetiology, histology, diagnosis and treatment. *J Laryngol Otol.* 1984;98:1237–1240.
5. Feder RJ, Michell MJ. Hyperfunctional, hyperacidic, and intubation granulomas. *Arch Otolaryngol.* 1984;110:582–584.
6. Belmont JR, Grundfast K. Congenital laryngeal stridor (laryngomalacia): etiologic factors and associated disorders. *Ann Otol Rhinol Laryngol.* 1984;93:430–437.
7. Olson NR. Effects of stomach acid on the larynx. *Proc Am Laryngol Assoc.* 1983;104:108–112.
8. Ohman L, Olofsson J, Tibbling L, Ericsson G. Esophageal dysfunction in patients with contact ulcer of the larynx. *Ann Otol Rhinol Laryngol.* 1983;92:228–230.
9. Bain WM, Harrington JW, Thomas LE, Schaefer SD. Head and neck manifestations of gastroesophageal reflux. *Laryngoscope.* 1983;93:175–179.
10. Orenstein SR, Orenstein DM, Whitington PF. Gastroesophageal reflux causing stridor. *Chest.* 1983;84:301–302.
11. Ward PH, Berci G. Observations on the pathogenesis of chronic nonspecific pharyngitis and laryngitis. *Laryngoscope.* 1982;92:1377–1382.

12. Ward PH, Zwitman D, Hanson D, Berci G. Contact ulcers and granulomas of the larynx: new insights into their etiology as a basis for more rational treatment. *Otolaryngol Head Neck Surg.* 1980; 88:262–269.

13. Goldberg M, Noyek AM, Pritzker KP. Laryngeal granuloma secondary to gastroesophageal reflux. *J Otolaryngol.* 1978;7:196–202.

14. Chodosh PL. Gastro-esophago-pharyngeal reflux. *Laryngoscope.* 1977;87:1418–1427.

15. Toohill RJ, Kuhn JC. Role of refluxed acid in pathogenesis of laryngeal disorders. *Am J Med.* 1997;103(suppl 5A):100S–106S.

16. Wiener GJ, Koufman JA, Wu WC, et al. Chronic hoarseness secondary to gastroesophageal reflux disease: documentation with 24-hr ambulatory pH monitoring. *Am J Gastroenterol.* 1989;84:1503–1508.

17. Sataloff RT, Spiegel JR, Hawkshaw MJ. Strobovideolaryngoscopy: results and clinical value. *Ann Otol Rhinol Laryngol.* 1991;100:725–727.

18. Koufman JA, Wiener GJ, Wu WC, Castell DO. Reflux laryngitis and its sequelae: the diagnostic role of ambulatory 24-hour pH monitoring. *J Voice.* 1988;2:78–89.

19. Toohill RJ, Ulualp SO, Shaker R. Evaluation of gastroesophageal reflux in patients with laryngotracheal stenosis. *Ann Otol Rhinol Laryngol.* 1998;107:1010–1014.

20. Ross JA, Noordzji JP, Woo P. Voice disorders in patients with suspected laryngo-pharyngeal reflux disease. *J Voice.* 1998;12:84–88.

21. Rothstein SG. Reflux and vocal disorders in singers with bulimia. *J Voice.* 1988;12:89–90.

22. Kuhn J, Toohill RJ, Ulualp SO, et al. Pharyngeal acid reflux events in patients with vocal cord nodules. *Laryngoscope.* 1998;108:1146–1149.

23. Gumpert L, Kalach N, Dupont C, Contencin P. Hoarseness and gastroesophageal reflux in children. *J Laryngol Otol.* 1998;112:49–54.

24. Halstead LA. Role of gastroesophageal reflux in pediatric upper airway disorders. *Otolaryngol Head Neck Surg.* 1999;120:208–214.

25. Al-Sabbagh G, Wo JM. Supraesophageal manifestations of gastroesophageal reflux disease. *Semin Gastrointest Dis.* 1999;10:113–119.

26. Hanson DG, Jiang JJ. Diagnosis and management of chronic laryngitis associated with reflux. *Am J Med.* 2000;108(suppl 4a):112S–119S.

27. Grontved AM, West F. pH monitoring in patients with benign voice disorders. *Acta Otolaryngol Suppl.* 2000;543:229–231.

28. Koufman JA, Amin MR, Panetti M. Prevalence of reflux in 113 consecutive patients with laryngeal and voice disorders. *Otolaryngol Head Neck Surg.* 2000;123:385–388.

29. Poelmans J, Tack J, Feenstra L. Chronic middle ear disease and gastroesophageal reflux disease: a causal relation? *Otol Neurotol.* 2001;22:447–450.

30. Tasker A, Dettmar PW, Panetti M, et al. Reflux of gastric juice and glue ear in children. *Lancet.* 2002;359:493. Letter.

31. Loehrl TA, Smith TL, Darling RJ, et al. Autonomic dysfunction, vasomotor rhinitis, and extraesophageal manifestations of gastroesophageal reflux. *Otolaryngol Head Neck Surg.* 2002;126:382–387.

32. Koufman JA. The otolaryngologic manifestations of gastroesophageal reflux disease (GERD): a clinical investigation of 225 patients using ambulatory 24-hour pH monitoring and an experimental investigation of the role of acid and pepsin in the development of laryngeal injury. *Laryngoscope.* 1991;101(suppl 53):1–78.

33. Sataloff RT. *Professional Voice: The Science and Art of Clinical Care.* 3rd ed. San Diego, CA: Singular Publishing Group; 2005.

34. Rosen DC, Sataloff RT. *The Psychology of Voice Disorders.* San Diego, CA: Singular Publishing Group; 1997.

2

Anatomy and Physiology of the Voice

The anatomic and physiologic basis for many symptoms of laryngopharyngeal reflux (LPR) seems fairly obvious initially. Topical irritation, muscle spasm, bronchospasm occurring in response to acidic aspiration, halitosis, sore throat, and other symptoms are easy to understand, although some have unexpectedly complex physiology. In addition, vagal reflexes triggered by distal esophageal acid irritation may cause events and responses that affect the voice even without having acid contact the larynx. Regardless of the mechanism, the effects of reflux laryngitis on voice function are often greater than might be anticipated on the basis of physical findings. To understand the impact of reflux disease on phonation, it is helpful to review current concepts in anatomy and physiology of the voice. Naturally, the physiology of phonation is much more complex than this brief chapter might imply. The reader interested in acquiring more than a clinically essential introduction to the voice is encouraged to consult other literature, including Sundberg's excellent text, *The Science of the Singing Voice*,[1] an overview of the mechanics of phonation by Scherer,[2] Sataloff's *Professional Voice: The Science and Art of Clinical Care* (third edition),[3] and the numerous references and suggested readings compiled in these sources.

ANATOMY

The *larynx* is essential to voice production, but the anatomy of the voice is not limited to the larynx. The vocal mechanism includes the abdominal and back musculature, rib cage, lungs, pharynx, oral cavity, and nose. Each component performs an important function in voice production, although it is possible to produce voice even without a larynx—for example, in patients who have undergone laryngectomy. In addition, virtually all parts of the body play some role in voice production and may be responsible for voice dysfunction. Even a pathologic condition as remote as a sprained ankle, by altering the standing posture, may impair abdominal, back, and thoracic muscle function, resulting in vocal inefficiency, weakness, fatigue, and hoarseness.

The larynx is composed of 4 basic anatomic units: the skeleton, intrinsic muscles, extrinsic muscles, and mucosa. The most important parts of the laryngeal skeleton are the thyroid cartilage, cricoid cartilage, and 2 arytenoid cartilages (Figure 2–1). Intrinsic muscles of the larynx are connected to these cartilages (Figure 2–2). One of the intrinsic muscles, the thyroarytenoid or vocalis muscle, extends on each side from the arytenoid cartilage to the inside of the thyroid cartilage just below and

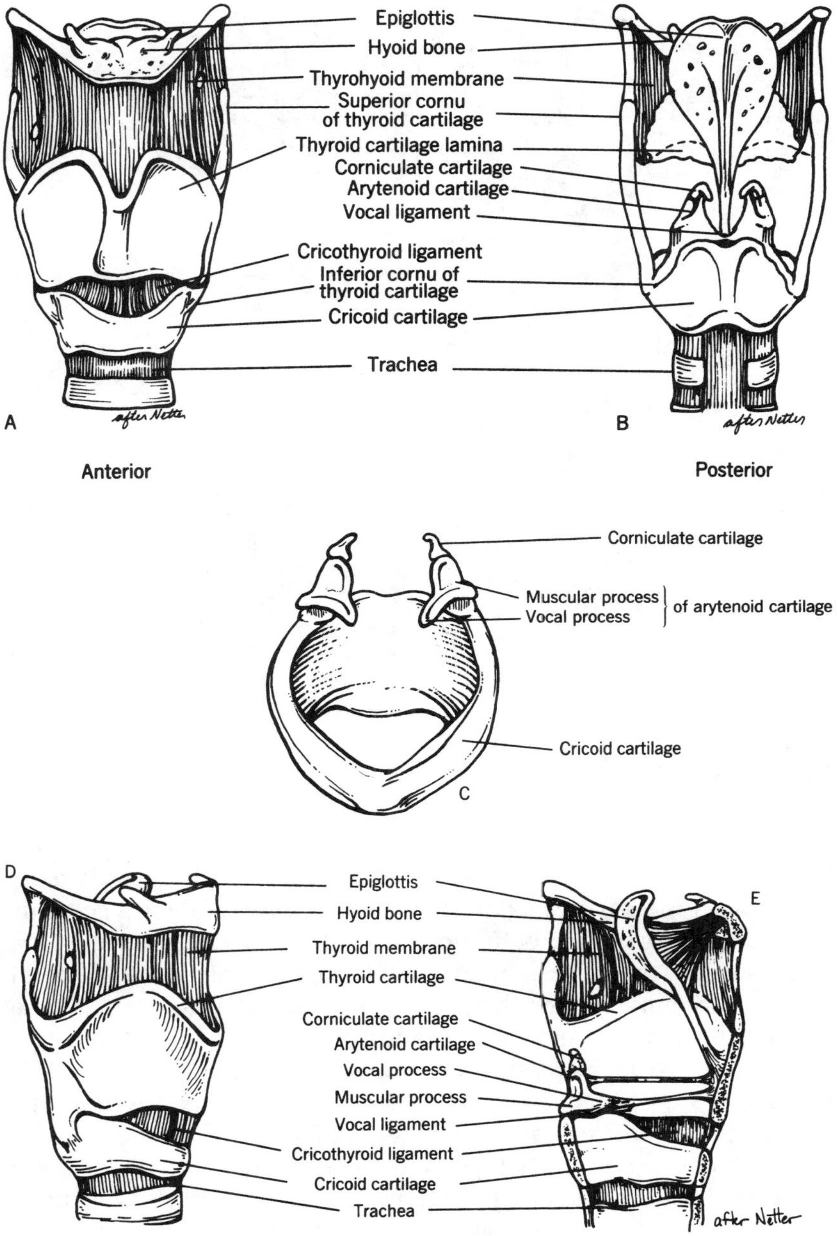

Figure 2–1. Cartilages of the larynx.

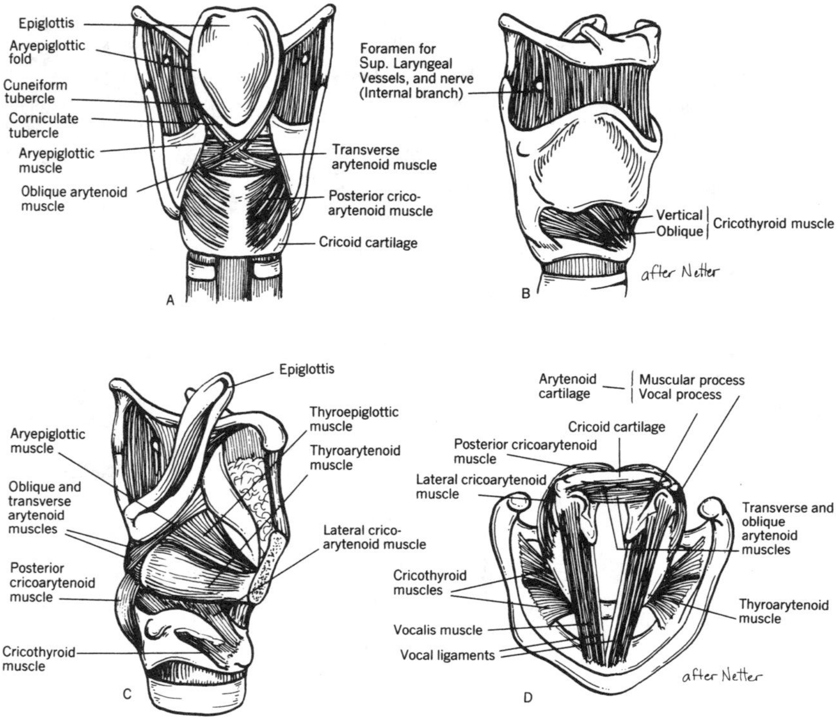

Figure 2–2. Intrinsic muscles of the larynx.

behind the "Adam's apple"; these paired muscles form the body of the vocal folds (popularly called the vocal cords). The vocal folds act as the oscillator or voice source of the vocal tract. The space between the vocal folds is called the glottis and is used as an anatomic reference point. The intrinsic muscles alter the position, shape, and tension of the vocal folds by bringing them together (adduction) or apart (abduction) or by stretching them, increasing longitudinal tension (Figure 2–3). These alterations are possible because the laryngeal cartilages are connected by soft attachments that allow changes in their relative angles and distances, with consequent changes in the shape and tension of the tissues suspended between them. The arytenoid cartilages are also capable of rocking, rotating, and gliding, permitting complex vocal fold motion and alteration in the shape of the vocal fold edge (Figure 2–4). All but 1 of the muscles on each side of the larynx are innervated by 1 of the 2 recurrent laryngeal nerves (RLNs).

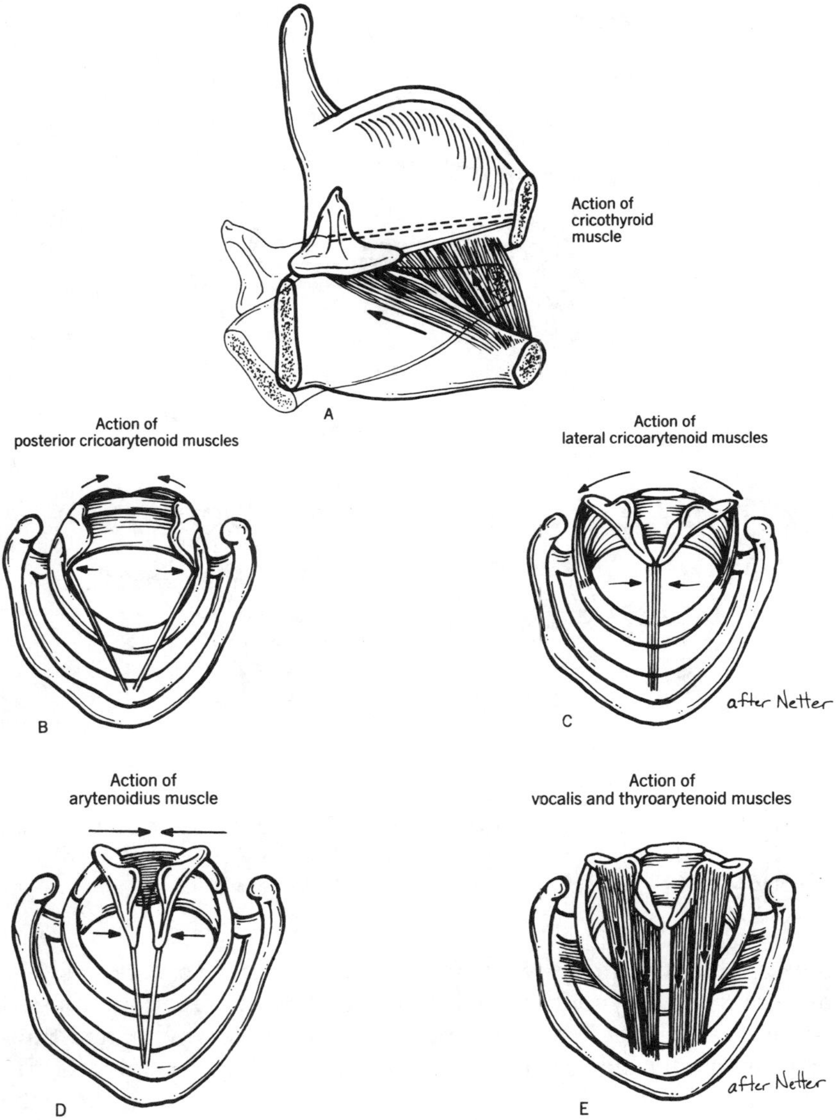

Figure 2–3. Action of the intrinsic muscles.

Because the RLN structure runs a long course from the neck down into the chest and then back up to the larynx (hence the name "recurrent"), it is easily injured (stretched or severed) by trauma or during

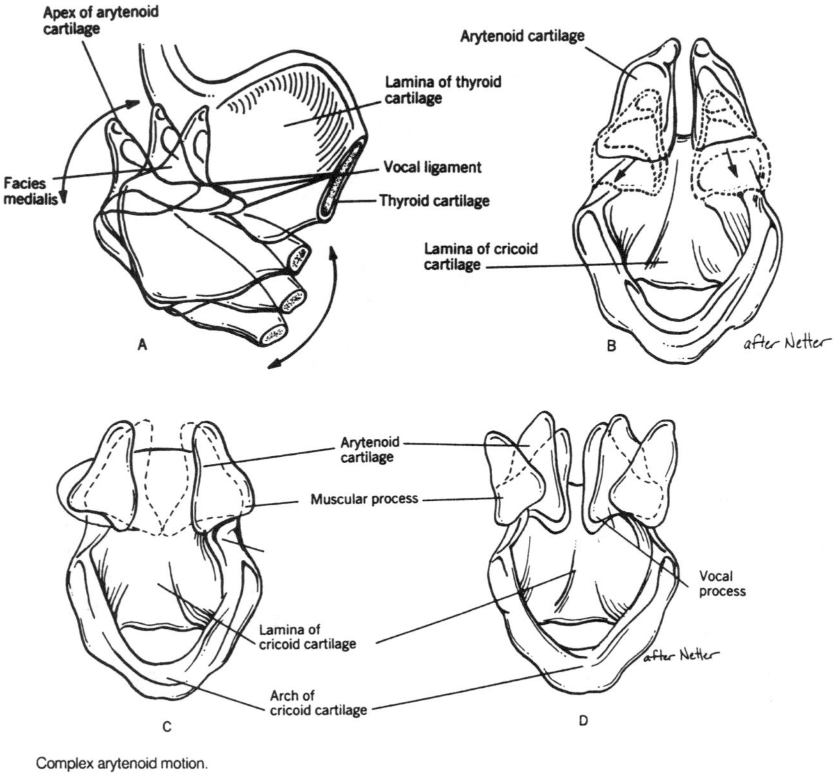

Figure 2–4. Complex arytenoid motion. (Originally published in Gould WJ, Sataloff RT, Spiegel JR. *Voice Surgery*. St Louis, MO: Mosby-Yearbook; 1993:164.)

neck and chest surgery, which may result in vocal fold paralysis. The remaining cricothyroid muscle is innervated by the superior laryngeal nerve on each side, which is especially susceptible to viral and traumatic injury. It produces increases in longitudinal tension important in volume and pitch control. The "false vocal folds" are located above the vocal folds and, unlike the true vocal folds, do not make contact during normal speaking or singing. The neuroanatomy and neurophysiology of phonation are exceedingly complicated and only partly understood. As the new field of neurolaryngology advances, a more thorough understanding of the subject will become increasingly important to the clinician. The reader interested in acquiring a deeper, scientific understanding of neurolaryngology is encouraged to consult the growing literature on this subject, particularly a fine, well-referenced review by Garrett and Larson.[4]

Because the attachments of the laryngeal cartilages are flexible, the positions of the cartilages with respect to each other change when the laryngeal skeleton is elevated or lowered. Such changes in vertical height are controlled by the extrinsic laryngeal muscles, or strap muscles of the neck. When the angles and distances between cartilages change because of this accordion effect, the resting length of the intrinsic muscles is changed as a consequence. Such large adjustments in intrinsic muscles interfere with fine control of smooth vocal quality. For this reason, classically trained singers are generally taught to use their extrinsic muscles to maintain the laryngeal skeleton at a relatively constant height regardless of pitch. That is, they learn to avoid the natural tendency of the larynx to rise with ascending pitch and to fall with descending pitch, thereby enhancing uniform quality throughout the vocal range.

The soft tissues lining the larynx are also much more complex than was originally thought. The mucosa forms the thin, lubricated surfaces of the vocal folds that make contact when the vocal folds are closed. It has the same appearance as that of the mucosa lining the inside of the mouth. Throughout most of the larynx, there are goblet cells and pseudostratified ciliated columnar epithelium designed for handling mucous secretions, similar to mucosa found throughout the respiratory tract. However, the mucosa overlying the vocal folds themselves is different. First, it is stratified squamous epithelium, better suited to withstand the trauma of vocal fold contact. Second, the vocal fold is not simply muscle covered with mucosa; rather, it consists of 5 layers, as described by Hirano.[5] He points out that mechanically, the vocal fold structures act more like 3 layers, consisting of the *cover* (epithelium and superficial layer of the lamina propria), the *transition layer* (intermediate and deep layers of the lamina propria), and the *body* (the vocalis muscle). It is essential for surgeons to appreciate this anatomy and to understand the importance of preserving it during surgical intervention.

The *supraglottic vocal tract* includes the pharynx, tongue, palate, oral cavity, nose, and other structures. Together, they act as a resonator and are largely responsible for vocal quality or timbre and the perceived character of all speech sounds. The vocal folds themselves produce only a "buzzing" sound. During the course of vocal training for singing, acting, or professional speaking, changes occur not only in the larynx but also in the motion, control, and shape of the supraglottic vocal tract.

The *infraglottic vocal tract* serves as the *power source* for the voice. Singers and actors refer to the entire power source complex as their "support" or "diaphragm." Actually, the anatomy of support for phonation is especially complicated and not completely understood. Nevertheless, it is quite important because deficiencies in support are frequently responsible for voice dysfunction.

The purpose of the support mechanism is to generate a force that directs a controlled airstream between the vocal folds. Active respiratory forces work in concert with passive forces. The principal muscles of inspiration are the diaphragm (a dome-shaped muscle that extends along the bottom of the rib cage) and the external intercostal muscles. During quiet respiration, expiration is largely passive. The lungs and rib cage generate passive expiratory forces in many common circumstances, such as after a full breath.

Many of the muscles used for active expiration are also employed in support for phonation. Muscles of active expiration either raise the intra-abdominal pressure, forcing the diaphragm upward, or lower the ribs or sternum to decrease the dimensions of the thorax, or both, thereby compressing air in the chest. The primary muscles of expiration are the "abdominal muscles," but the internal intercostals and other chest and back muscles are also involved. Trauma or surgery that alters the structure or function of these muscles or ribs undermines the power source of the voice, as do diseases that impair expiration, such as asthma. Deficiencies in the support mechanism often result in compensatory efforts that utilize the laryngeal muscles, which are not designed for power source functions. Such behaviors can result in decreased vocal fold function, rapid voice fatigue, pain, and even structural pathology including vocal fold nodules. Current expert treatment for such problems focuses on correction of the underlying malfunction rather than on surgery.

PHYSIOLOGY OF THE VOICE

The physiology of voice production is complex. Volitional production of voice begins in the cerebral cortex (Figure 2–5). The command for vocalization involves complex interaction among centers for speech and other areas. For singing, speech directives must be integrated with information from the brain's centers for musical and artistic expression. The "idea" of the planned vocalization is conveyed to the precentral gyrus in the motor cortex, which transmits another set of instructions to the motor nuclei in the brainstem and spinal cord. These areas send out the complicated messages necessary for coordinated activity of the laryngeal, thoracic, and abdominal musculature and the vocal tract

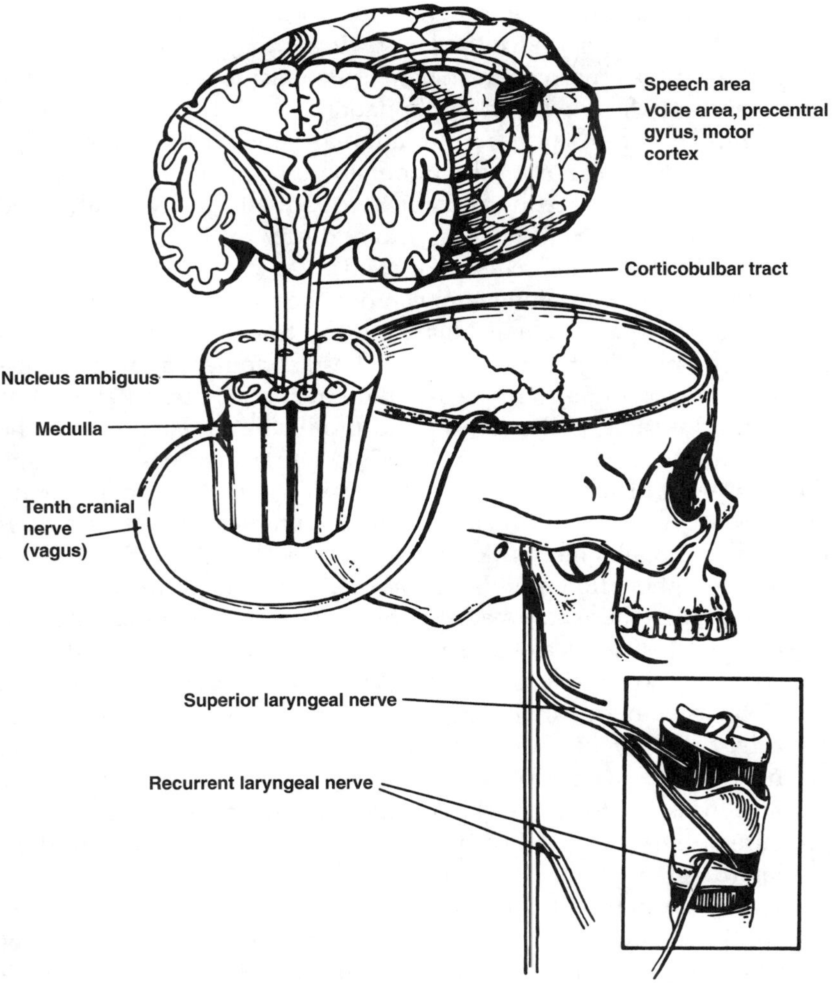

Figure 2–5. Simplified summary of pathway for volitional phonation. (Originally published in Gould WJ, Sataloff RT, Spiegel JR. *Voice Surgery*. St Louis, MO: Mosby-Yearbook; 1993:166.)

articulators. Additional refinement of motor activity is provided by the extrapyramidal and autonomic nervous systems. These impulses combine to produce a sound that is transmitted to not only the ears of the listener(s) but also to those of the speaker or singer. Auditory feedback is transmitted from the ear through the brainstem to the cerebral cortex, and adjustments are made to permit the vocalist to match the sound produced with the sound intended, taking into account the acoustic properties of the environment. There is also tactile feedback from the throat and muscles involved in phonation, which is believed to help in the fine-tuning of vocal output, although the mechanism and role of tactile feedback are not fully understood. In many trained singers and speakers, the ability to use tactile feedback effectively is cultivated because of expected interference with auditory feedback by ancillary noise such as that of an orchestra or band.

Phonation requires interaction among the power source, oscillator, and resonator. The voice may be likened to a brass instrument, such as a trumpet. Power is generated by the chest, abdomen, and back musculature, producing a high-pressure airstream. The trumpeter's lips open and close against the mouthpiece, producing a buzz similar to the sound produced by the vocal folds. This sound then passes through the trumpet, which has resonance characteristics that shape the sound we associate with trumpet music. The nonmouthpiece portion of a brass instrument is analogous to the supraglottic vocal tract.

During phonation, rapid, complex adjustments of the infraglottic musculature are necessary because the resistance changes almost continuously as the glottis closes, opens, and changes shape. At the beginning of each phonatory cycle, the vocal folds are approximated. That is, the glottis is obliterated. This permits infraglottic pressure to build up, typically to a level of about 7 cm of water for conversational speech. At this point, the vocal folds are convergent (Figure 2–6, diagram 1). Because the vocal folds are closed, there is no airflow. The subglottic pressure pushes the vocal folds progressively farther apart from the bottom up (diagrams 1 and 2), until a space develops (diagram 3) and air begins to flow. Bernoulli force is created by the air that passes between the vocal folds; this force combines with the mechanical properties of the folds to begin closing the lower portion of the glottis almost immediately (diagrams 4 through 7), even while the upper edges are still separating. The upper portion of the vocal folds has strong elastic properties, which tend to make the vocal folds snap back to the midline. This force becomes more dominant as the upper edges are stretched farther apart and as the force of the airstream diminishes because of approximation of the lower edges of the vocal folds. Therefore, the upper portions of the vocal folds return to the midline (diagrams 8 and 9), completing the glottic cycle. Subglottic pressure then builds again (diagram 10), and the events are repeated. The frequency of vibration (number of cycles of openings and closings per second, measured in hertz [Hz]) is dependent

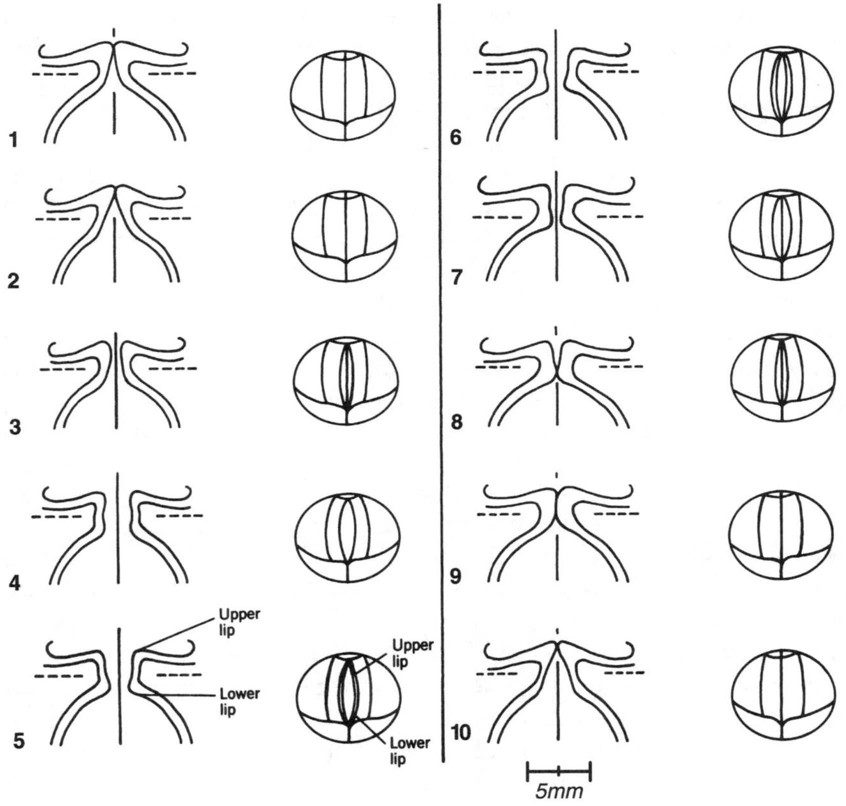

Figure 2–6. Frontal view (*left*) and view from above (*right*) illustrating the normal pattern of vocal fold vibration. The vocal folds close and open the glottis from the inferior aspect of the vibratory margin upward. (From Hirano M. *Clinical Examination of the Voice*. New York, NY: Springer-Verlag; 1981:44, with permission.)

on the air pressure and mechanical properties of the vocal folds, which are regulated by the laryngeal muscles.

Frequency corresponds closely with our perception of pitch. Under most circumstances, as the vocal folds are thinned and stretched, and air pressure is increased, the frequency of air pulse emission increases, and pitch goes up. In understanding this myoelastic-aerodynamic mechanism of phonation, it is important to note not only that the vocal folds emit pulses of air, rather than vibrating like strings, but also that there is a vertical phase difference. That is, the lower portion of the vocal folds begins to open and close before the upper portion. The rippling displacement of the vocal fold cover produces a mucosal wave that can be examined clinically under stroboscopic light. If this complex motion is impaired, hoarseness or other changes in voice quality may result.

The sound produced by the vibrating vocal folds (voice source signal) is a complex tone containing a fundamental frequency (see below) and many overtones, or higher harmonic partials. The amplitude of the partials decreases uniformly at approximately 12 decibels (dB) per octave. It is of interest that the spectrum of the voice source is about the same in ordinary speakers as it is in singers and trained speakers. However, voice quality differences occur as the voice source signal passes through the supraglottic vocal tract (Figure 2–7).

The pharynx, oral cavity, and nasal cavity act as a series of interconnected resonators, more complex than a trumpet or other single resonators. As with other resonators, some frequencies are attenuated, whereas others are enhanced. Enhanced frequencies are radiated with higher relative amplitudes. Sundberg[1] has shown that the vocal tract has 4 or 5 important resonance frequencies called *formants*. The presence of formants alters the uniformly sloping voice source spectrum, creating peaks at formant frequencies. These alterations of the voice source spectral envelope are responsible for distinguishable sounds of speech and song. Formant frequencies are established by vocal tract shape, which can be altered by laryngeal, pharyngeal, and oral cavity musculature. Although overall vocal tract length and shape are individually fixed and determined by age and gender (women and children have shorter vocal tracts and higher formant frequencies than males), mastering adjustment of vocal tract shape is fundamental to voice training. Although the formants differ for different vowels, one resonant frequency, known as the "singer formant," has received particular attention. The singer formant occurs in the vicinity of 2300 to 3200 Hz for all vowel spectra and appears to be responsible for the "ring" in a singer's or trained speaker's voice. The audibility and clarity of a trained voice heard even over a loud choir or orchestra are dependent primarily on the presence of the singer formant.[1]

Of interest, there is little or no significant difference in maximum vocal intensity between a trained and a nontrained singer. The singer formant also contributes significantly to the difference in timbre among voice categories, occurring in basses at about 2400 Hz, baritones at 2600 Hz, tenors at 2800 Hz, mezzo-sopranos at 2900 Hz, and sopranos at 3200 Hz. It is frequently much less prominent in high soprano singing.

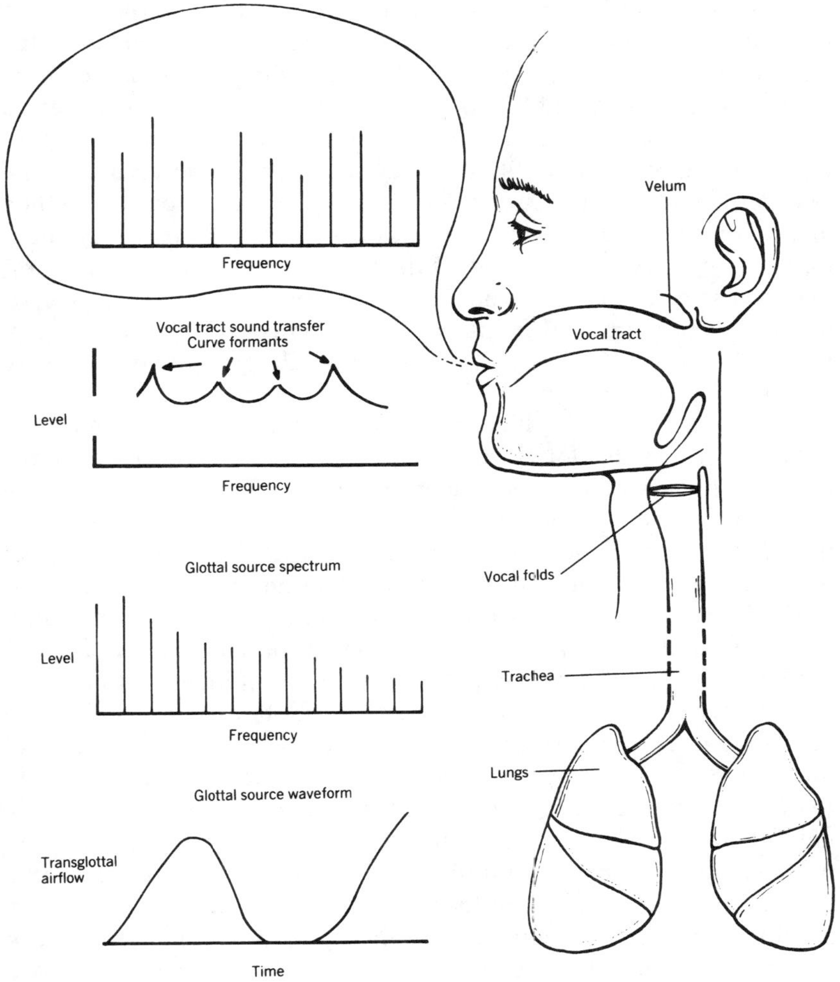

Figure 2-7. Determinants of the spectrum of a vowel (oral-output signal). (From Sataloff R. *Professional Voice: The Science and Art of Clinical Care.* 3rd ed. San Diego, CA: Plural Publishing; 2005:276, with permission.)

Control mechanisms for 2 vocal characteristics are particularly important: fundamental frequency and intensity. *Fundamental frequency,* which corresponds to pitch, can be altered by changing either the air pressure or the mechanical properties of the vocal folds, although the latter is more efficient under most conditions. Contracting the cricothyroid muscle makes the thyroid cartilage pivot, thereby increasing the distance between the thyroid and arytenoid cartilages and consequently stretching the vocal folds. This increases the surface area exposed to subglottic pressure and makes the air pressure more effective in opening the vocal folds. In addition, the elastic fibers of the vocal fold are stretched, making them more efficient at snapping back together. Hence, the cycles shorten and repeat more frequently, and the fundamental frequency and pitch rise. Other muscles, including the thyroarytenoid, also contribute. Raising the pressure of the airstream also tends to increase fundamental frequency, a phenomenon for which singers must compensate. Otherwise, their pitch would go up whenever they tried to sing more loudly.

Vocal *intensity*, which corresponds to loudness, depends on the degree to which the glottal wave excites the air in the vocal tract. Raising the air pressure creates greater amplitude of vocal fold vibration and, consequently, increased vocal intensity. However, it is actually not the vibrating vocal fold but rather the sudden cessation of airflow that is responsible for establishing acoustic vibration in the vocal tract and controlling intensity. This mechanism is similar to that in acoustic vibration from hand clapping. In the larynx, the sharper the flow cutoff is, the more intense the sounds are. In fact, greater vocal intensity is marked primarily by a steeper closing phase of the glottal wave, achieved by both higher air pressure and biomechanical vocal fold changes that increase glottal resistance to airflow. Assessing an individual's ability to optimize adjustments of air pressure and glottal resistance may be helpful in identifying and correcting voice dysfunction. If high subglottic pressure is combined with high adductory vocal fold force, glottal airflow and the amplitude of the voice source fundamental frequency are low. This type of phonation is called pressed phonation and can be measured clinically with the use of flow glottography. Flow glottography employs inverse filtering of the supraglottic contribution to voice in order to generate a wave that defines voice source signal characteristics. The flow glottogram wave amplitude indicates the type of phonation being used, and the slope (closing rate) provides information about the sound pressure level or loudness. If adductory forces are so weak that the vocal folds do not make contact, the glottis becomes inefficient and the voice source fundamental is also low. This type of phonation is known as breathy phonation. Flow phonation is characterized by lower subglottic pressure and lower adductory force. These conditions increase the dominance of the fundamental frequency of the voice source. Sundberg has shown that the amplitude of the fundamental frequency can be increased by 15 dB or more in changing from pressed phonation to flow phonation.[1(p80)] If a patient habitually uses pressed phonation, considerable effort will be required to achieve loud voicing. The muscle patterns and force used to compensate for this laryngeal inefficiency may cause vocal damage.

REFERENCES

1. Sundberg J. *The Science of the Singing Voice.* DeKalb, IL: Northern Illinois University Press; 1987.
2. Scherer RS. Physiology of phonation: a review of basic mechanics. In: Ford CN, Bless DM, eds. *Phonosurgery.* New York, NY: Raven Press; 1991:77–93.
3. Sataloff RT. *Professional Voice: The Science and Art of Clinical Care.* 3rd ed. San Diego, CA: Plural Publishing; 2005.
4. Garrett JD, Larson CR. Neurology of the laryngeal system. In: Ford CN, Bless DM, eds. *Phonosurgery.* New York, NY: Raven Press; 1991: 43–76.
5. Hirano M. Phonosurgery. Basic and clinical investigations. *Otologia (Fukuoka).* 1975;21:239–442.

3

Anatomy and Physiology of the Esophagus and Its Sphincters

ANATOMY

The human esophagus is a muscular tube whose major function is transport of food from the mouth to the stomach.[1] It is bounded by 2 tonically contracted circular muscle sphincters, 1 at each end. The median length of the esophageal body, between the 2 sphincters, is 22 cm in adult females and 24 cm in adult males. Individual variations in length are normally distributed in both genders[1] (Figure 3–1). The upper esophageal sphincter (UES) consists primarily of the striated muscle of the cricopharyngeus muscle but is enhanced by the inferior pharyngeal constrictors and the circular muscles of the upper esophagus. Because of the anterior attachment of the cricopharyngeus to the cricoid cartilage of the larynx, the strongest contractile force of this sphincter occurs in the anterior-posterior direction, producing a slitlike configuration with the widest portion facing laterally.[2] The UES, like the striated musculature of the tongue, pharynx, and upper portion of the esophagus, is innervated as for skeletal muscle, receiving motor input directly from the brainstem (nucleus ambiguus) to the motor end-plates in the muscle. Tonicity is maintained by continuous stimulation, which is temporarily inhibited during a swallow.

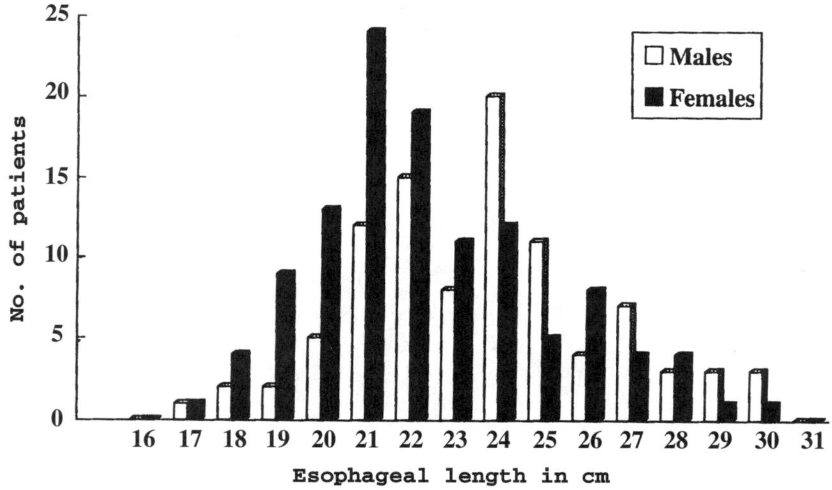

Figure 3–1. Distribution of esophageal length in 212 patients and normal volunteers. Approximation to a normal distribution is verified by similar means and medians (males: mean = 23.6 cm, median = 24.0 cm; females: mean = 22.4 cm, median = 22.0 cm).

The lower esophageal sphincter (LES), like most of the gastrointestinal (GI) tract, consists entirely of smooth muscle. This sphincter is much more rounded in its closure, yet still demonstrates some degree of radial asymmetry, with the highest pressures in the posterolateral direction.[3] Innervation of the LES originates from the dorsal motor nucleus of the brainstem, and the efferent fibers are carried through the vagus nerve and synapse in the myenteric plexus in the region of the LES.

The muscular wall of the esophagus is composed of an inner circular and an outer longitudinal layer, with no serosa overlying the muscle layers. The UES and the upper portion of the tubular esophagus are primarily striated muscle. Recent studies have indicated that muscle occurs in the upper 4 to 5 cm of the human esophagus, although it is quite variable in different persons and in the different muscle layers. Consistently, more than half the length of the human esophagus at its distal end is entirely smooth muscle.[4] As in the LES, the smooth muscle portion of the tubular esophagus is innervated primarily via the vagus nerve by neurons arising in the dorsal motor nucleus connecting to the myenteric plexus.

PHYSIOLOGY

Swallowing, or deglutition, has 3 stages: the oral (voluntary) stage, the pharyngeal (involuntary) stage, and the esophageal stage. These 3 closely coordinated processes are regulated through the swallowing center in the medulla.[5]

Oral Stage

The first stage of deglutition is the oral stage. This preparatory stage includes mechanical disruption of the food and mixing with salivary bicarbonate and enzymes (amylase, lipase). It is an essential process by which the swallowing mechanism is primed. Ingested food is voluntarily moved posteriorly by pistonlike movements of the tongue muscles, forcing the food bolus toward the pharynx and pushing it backward and upward against the palate. Once the food has been delivered to the pharynx, the process becomes involuntary. The oral, preparatory stage obviously requires proper functioning of the striated muscles of the tongue and pharynx and is the stage of swallowing that is likely to be abnormal in patients with neurologic or skeletal muscle disease. Adequate mentation is also necessary.

Pharyngeal Stage

During the pharyngeal stage of swallowing, the food is passed from the pharynx, through the UES, and into the proximal esophagus. This involuntary process requires the finely tuned coordinated sequences of contraction and relaxation, resulting in transfer of the ingested material while protecting the airway. The presence of food in the pharynx stimulates sensory receptors, which send impulses to the swallowing center in the brainstem. The central nervous system then initiates a series of involuntary responses that include the following:

1. The soft palate is pulled upward and closes the posterior nares.
2. The palatopharyngeal folds are pulled medially, limiting the opening through the pharynx.
3. The vocal folds are closed and the epiglottis swings backward and down to close the larynx.
4. The larynx is pulled upward and forward by the muscles attached to the hyoid bone, stretching the opening of the esophagus and UES.
5. The UES relaxes. Active relaxation of the usually tonic cricopharyngeus is essential to permit the passive opening of the UES created by the movement of the larynx.
6. Peristaltic contraction of the constrictor muscles of the pharynx produces the force that propels food into the esophagus.

This sequence is a coordinated mechanism that includes impulses carried by 5 cranial nerves. Sensory information to the swallowing center is carried along cranial nerves V, VII, IX, and X. The motor responses from the swallowing center are carried along cranial nerves V, VII, IX, X, and XII and the ansa cervicalis (C-1 and C-2). This intricate process takes just over 1 second from start to finish and requires coordination of pharyngeal contraction and UES relaxation (Figure 3–2). The UES is open for only ~500 ms.

Esophageal Stage

The main function of the esophagus is to transport ingested material from the mouth to the stomach. This active process requires contraction of both the longitudinal and circular muscular layers of the tubular

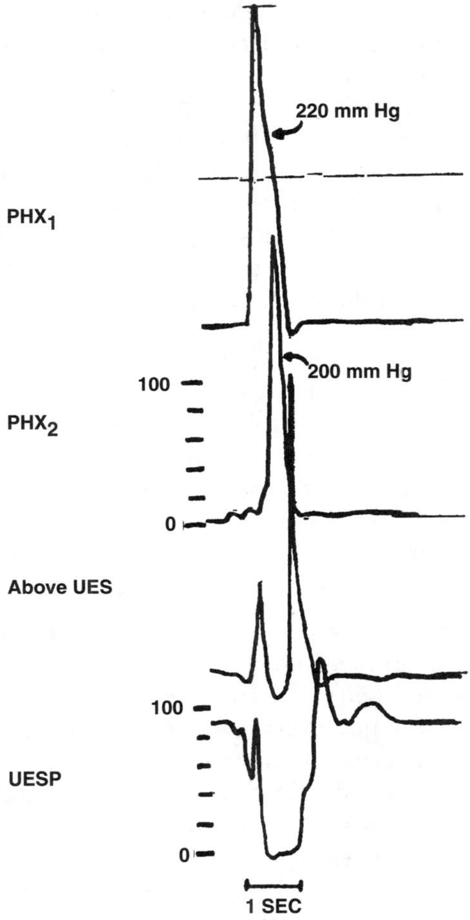

Figure 3–2. Motility tracing showing the coordinated sequence of contraction of the human pharynx and relaxation of the UES. The 4 recording sites are spaced at 3-cm intervals, with the lowest in the UES high-pressure zone (UESP), the second from the bottom located just proximal to the UES, and the next 2 sites at 3 cm (PHX 2) and 6 cm (PHX 1) farther proximal. The sequential contraction in the pharynx is noted in the 2 most proximal recording sites. The orad movement of the UES followed by UES relaxation and subsequent descent of the UES during the swallow generates the M configuration shown at the third recording site. The apparently longer UES "relaxation" seen in the distal sensor is an artifact produced by the orad movement of the sphincter away from the transducer during swallowing. The actual time of UES relaxation is ~0.5 seconds, as shown in the recording located second from the bottom.

esophagus and coordinated relaxation of the sphincters. At the onset of swallowing, the longitudinal muscle contracts, thereby shortening the esophagus to provide a structural base for the circular muscle contraction that forms the peristaltic wave. The sequential contraction of esophageal circular smooth muscle from proximal to distal generates the peristaltic clearing wave. (The neuromuscular control of this activity is described later.) Unlike other GI tract smooth muscle, the esophageal smooth muscle has a unique electrical activity pattern, showing only spiked potentials without underlying slow waves. Circular muscle contractions can be classified into 3 distinct patterns:

1. *Primary peristalsis.* This is the usual form of a contraction wave of circular muscle that progresses down the esophagus and is initiated by the central mechanisms that follow the voluntary act of swallowing. It follows sequentially the pressure generated in the pharynx and requires ~8 to 10 seconds to reach the distal esophagus. The LES relaxes at the onset of the swallow and remains relaxed until it contracts as a continuation of the progressive peristaltic wave. These pressure relationships are shown in Figure 3–3.
2. *Secondary peristalsis.* This represents a peristaltic contraction of the circular esophageal muscle, which begins without central stimulation. This is to say, it originates in the esophagus as a result of distention and usually continues until the esophagus is empty. Some food, particularly solid material, requires more than the single primary peristaltic wave for eventual clearance. This is accomplished by the secondary peristaltic waves. Thus, secondary peristalsis is the mechanism for clearing both ingested material and material that is refluxed from the stomach. Experimentally, secondary peristalsis can be demonstrated by inflating a balloon in the mid- to upper esophagus.
3. *Tertiary contractions.* This contraction pattern is identified primarily during barium x-ray studies of the esophagus. It represents a nonperistaltic series of contractile waves that appear as localized segmented indentations in the barium column. It has no known physiologic function.

One of the interesting phenomena seen in the esophagus occurs during the process of rapid sequential swallowing (≤10 seconds between successive voluntary swallows). This process results in inhibition of peristalsis, so-called deglutitive inhibition. Peristalsis is suspended during the continuation of a series of rapid swallows, and a large "clearing

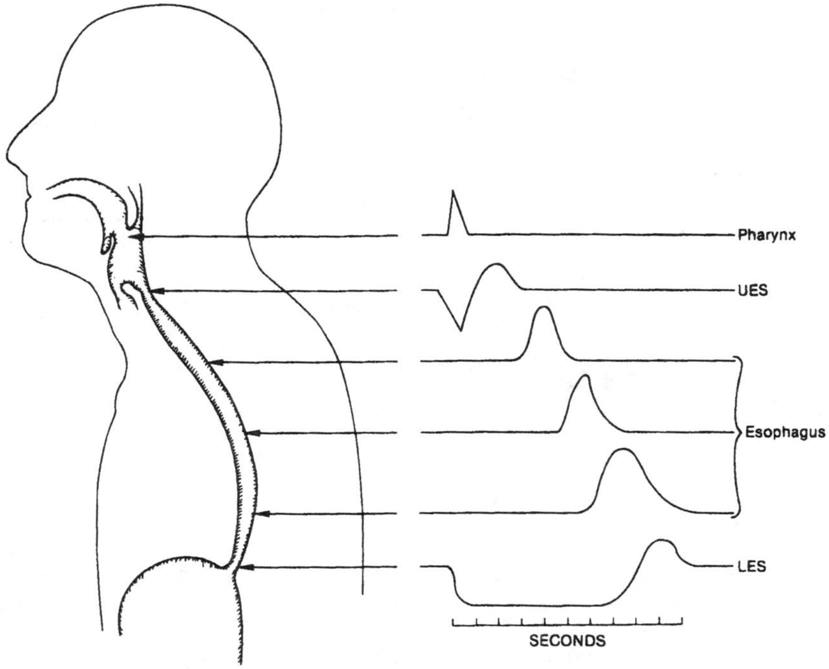

Figure 3-3. Schematic representation of the pressure sequence of a normal peristaltic wave. Note the pressure complex that begins in the pharynx and progressively closes off the UES and then moves sequentially down the esophageal body and closes the UES. Also note that LES relaxation begins with the onset of the swallow and continues until the peristaltic wave reaches the distal esophagus (8–10 seconds).

wave" occurs at the completion of the swallows (Figure 3–4). This phenomenon occurs because of the inhibitory neural discharge that arises from the central swallowing center during swallowing and because the esophageal musculature is refractory to further stimulation, which may persist for up to 10 seconds.[6]

IMPORTANCE OF THE SPHINCTERS

The esophagus is located in the thorax and has negative pressure relative to pressures in the pharynx proximally and the stomach distally.

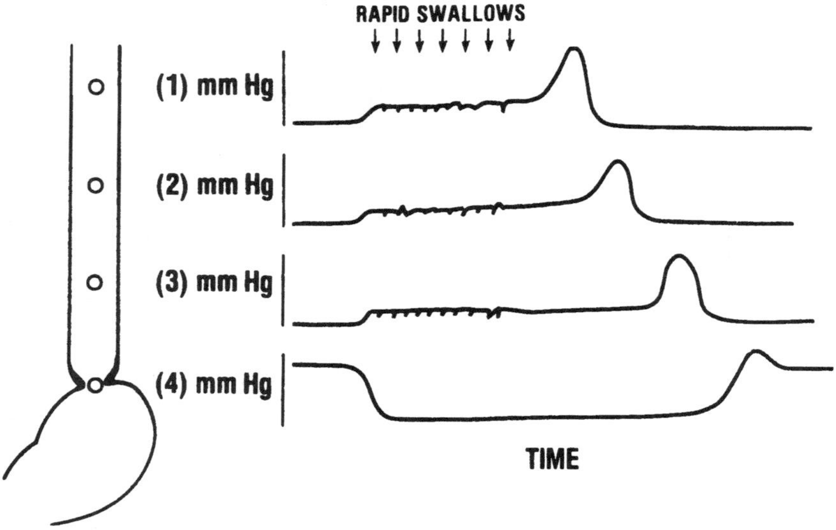

Figure 3-4. Demonstration of the phenomenon of deglutitive inhibition of the peristaltic sequence by rapid swallows separated by 5-second intervals. The LES remains relaxed throughout the sequence, as the esophageal body is inhibited from a peristaltic response until the termination of the swallow. At this point, the peristaltic clearing wave occurs.

Therefore, the sphincters must maintain constant closure to prevent abnormal movement of air or food into the esophagus. In the absence of a tonically contracted UES, air will flow freely into the esophagus during inspiration. In the presence of a weak LES, gastric contents are not inhibited from refluxing into the distal esophagus, particularly in the recumbent position. Pressure relationships in and around the esophagus and its sphincters are shown in Figure 3–5.

Upper Esophageal Sphincter

The UES maintains a constant closure, with its strongest forces acting in the anterior-posterior direction of the sling-shaped attachment of the cricopharyngeus to the cricoid cartilage. Normal pressures in the UES are ~100 mm Hg in the anterior-posterior direction and ~50 mm Hg laterally.[2]

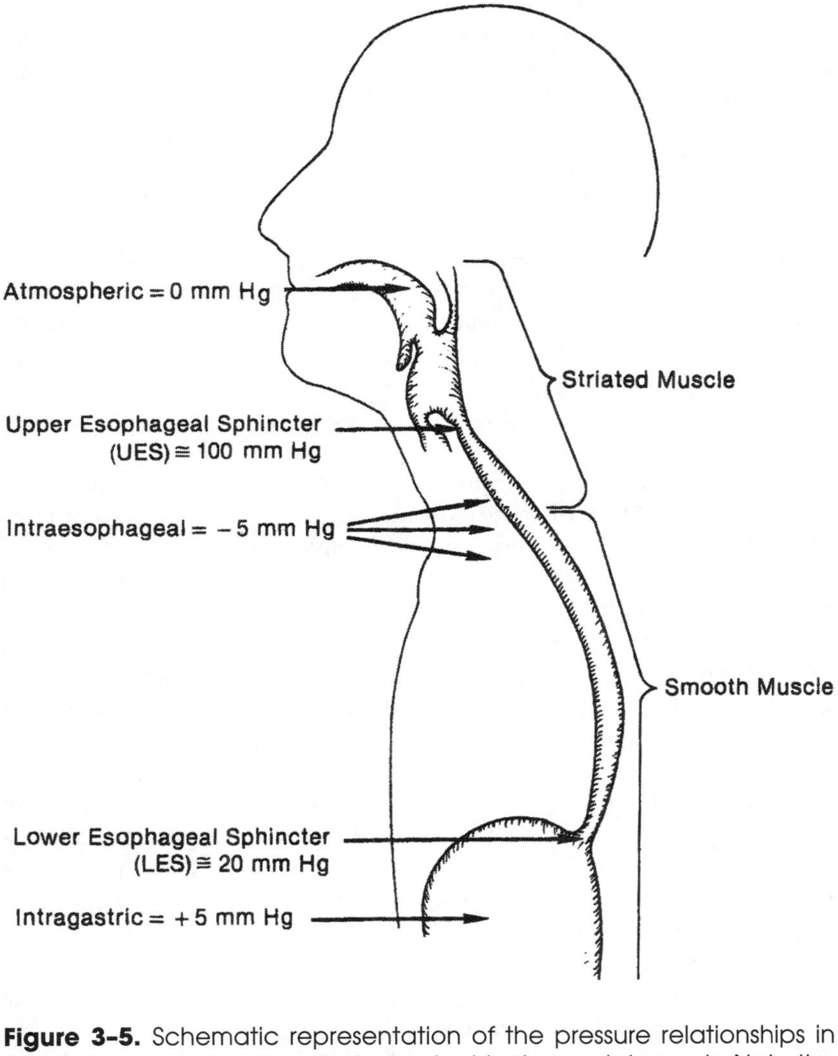

Figure 3–5. Schematic representation of the pressure relationships in the pharynx, esophagus, esophageal sphincter, and stomach. Note the negative intraesophageal pressure relative to both pharyngeal (atmospheric) pressure and intragastric pressure. This relationship underscores the importance of the sphincters in prevention of abnormal movement of fluids and air.

Lower Esophageal Sphincter

The tonically contracted LES normally maintains a closing pressure 10 to 45 mm Hg greater than the intragastric pressure below. By convention, LES pressure is measured as a gradient, in millimeters of mercury, higher than intragastric pressure, which is used as a zero reference. At the time of swallowing, the LES relaxes promptly in response to the initial neural discharge from the swallowing center in the brain and stays relaxed until the peristaltic wave reaches the end of the esophagus, producing sphincter closure. During relaxation, the pressure measured within the sphincter falls approximately to the level of gastric pressure and is considered a "complete" state of sphincter relaxation. Although there has been much controversy over the years, it is now generally accepted that the LES does not have to be located within the diaphragmatic crus to maintain a constant closing pressure. Thus, the presence of a sliding hiatal hernia is not necessarily detrimental to the physiologic function of this sphincter.

The LES maintains 2 important physiologic functions: the first is its role in prevention of gastroesophageal reflux, and the second is its ability to relax with swallowing to allow movement of ingested material into the stomach. The mechanism by which the circular smooth muscle of the LES maintains tonic closure has been a subject of considerable investigation over many years. At present, this mechanism is thought to be predominantly the result of intrinsic muscle activity, because investigations in animals have demonstrated that resting LES tone persists even after the destruction of all neural input by the neurotoxin tetrodotoxin.[7]

In addition, truncal vagotomy does not affect resting LES pressure in humans. Calcium channel–blocking agents, which exert their effect directly on the circular smooth muscle, produce decreases in LES pressures in animals and humans.[8,9] Also, some cholinergic tone appears to be present in many animal species and in humans, as an injection of atropine or botulinum toxin (Botox; Allergan, Irvine, CA) has been shown to produce marked decreases in resting LES pressure.[10,11]

The mechanism of relaxation of the LES in response to a swallow has also been a subject of considerable investigation and controversy. The precise neurotransmitter responsible for this response is not known. It is clear that this neurotransmitter is not a classic cholinergic or adrenergic agent because specific pharmacologic blockade of these mechanisms does not inhibit LES relaxation. This relaxation is a neural event, however, because it can be reproduced in animals by stimulation of the vagus nerve, and it is inhibited by tetrodotoxin.[12] The relationship among these maneuvers is summarized in Figure 3–6. Studies indicate

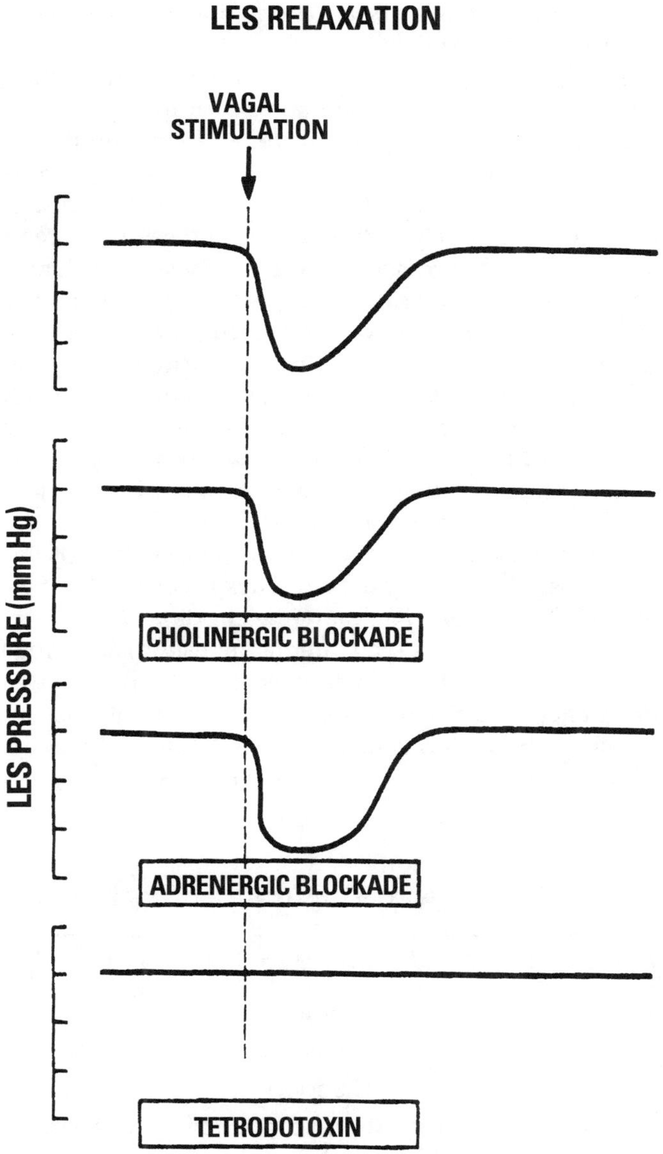

Figure 3-6. Summary of experiments on the neural regulation of LES relaxation in the opossum. Electrical stimulation of the vagus nerve produces relaxation, which is not inhibited by blocking either cholinergic or adrenergic pathways. However, the neural response is inhibited by the neurotoxin tetrodotoxin.

that the neurotransmitter may be a combination of vasoactive intestinal polypeptide and nitric oxide.[11,13]

The resting pressure of the LES is dynamic and demonstrates frequent changes. Measurement of pressures over long periods indicates that LES pressure varies considerably, even from minute to minute. Much of this variation is due to the effect of any of numerous factors that modulate pressure. These factors include foods ingested during meals and events such as cigarette smoking and gastric distention. The normal LES responds to transient increases in intra-abdominal pressure by raising its resting pressure to a greater degree than the pressure increases in the abdomen below. This normal protective mechanism guards against gastroesophageal reflux. In addition, many hormones and other peptide substances produced in the GI tract and in other areas of the body have been shown to affect LES pressure. These substances are summarized in Table 3–1. Many of these effects probably represent pharmacologic responses that have been shown to occur after intravenous injection or infusion of these substances in humans or animals. Whether they represent truly physiologic actions has not been clarified in most cases. The strongest candidates for physiologic hormonal control of the LES are cholecystokinin (the effects of which help explain the decrease in LES pressure seen after fat ingestion) and progesterone (the effects of which explain the decrease in LES pressure that occurs during pregnancy) . Finally, various neurotransmitters and pharmacologic agents have been shown to affect LES pressure. These agents are summarized in Table 3–2. The modulation of LES resting pressure is a

Table 3-1. Effects of Peptides and Hormones on LES Pressure

Increases LES	Decreases LES
Gastrin	Secretin
Motilin	Cholecystokinin
Substance P	Glucagon
Pancreatic polypeptide	Gastric inhibitory polypeptide (GIP)
Bombesin	Vasoactive intestinal polypeptide (VIP)
Leu-enkephalin	Pepside histidine isoleucine
Vasopressin	Progesterone
Angiotensin	

Table 3–2. Effects of Neurotransmitters and Pharmacologic Agents on LES Pressure

Increases LES	Decreases LES
Cholinergic (bethanechol) (α-adrenergic)	Nitric oxide
Metoclopramide	Dopamine (β-adrenergic)
Cisapride	Atropine
Calcium channel-blockers	Nitrates
Morphine	
Diazepam	
Theophylline	

complex mechanism that involves the interaction of the LES smooth muscle, neural control, and humoral factors.[14] Additional discussion of the LES can be found in Chapter 4.

Control of Esophageal Peristalsis

As noted previously, esophageal peristalsis is controlled via afferent and efferent neural connections through the swallowing center in the medulla. This central mechanism regulates the involuntary sequence of muscular events that occurs during swallowing and simultaneously inhibits the respiratory center in the medulla so that respiration is stopped during the pharyngeal stage of swallowing.

The direct innervation to the striated muscle of the pharynx and upper esophagus is carried via fibers from the brainstem (nucleus ambiguus) through the vagus nerve. The innervation of the smooth muscle of the distal esophagus and LES arises from the dorsal motor nucleus of the vagus and is carried through cholinergic visceral motor nerves to ganglia in the myenteric (Auerbach) plexus. Noncholinergic, nonadrenergic inhibitory nerves are also carried within the vagus.

The myenteric plexus in the esophageal portion of the enteric nervous system (the "brain in the gut") receives efferent impulses from the central nervous system and sensory afferents from the esophagus. Thus, impulses travel in 2 directions through this modulating area, which interconnects and regulates signals that result in normal peristalsis in the smooth muscle of the esophagus. One manifestation of the afferent control is the regulation of peristaltic squeezing pressures, to some degree, by the size of the ingested bolus. In addition, dry swallows often fail to provide adequate stimulation for the action of the myenteric plexus as the primary regulatory mechanism of esophageal peristalsis in the smooth muscle portion, as shown by observations that bilateral cervical vagotomy in animals does not abolish peristalsis in this area.

Interesting results have been obtained from in vitro studies of esophageal smooth muscle preparations.[15] Using muscle from the opossum esophagus, it has been shown that the longitudinal smooth muscle demonstrates a sustained contraction during electrical field stimulation; this phenomenon is called the duration response. This response is neural and cholinergic because it can be blocked with both atropine and tetrodotoxin. The circular smooth muscle of the opossum esophagus shows a quite different response. With the onset of electrical stimulation, there is a brief, small contraction at the beginning of the stimulus, known as the "on response." This response is quite variable and has no known physiologic role. The on response is followed by a much larger contraction that occurs after the termination of the stimulus, known as the "off response." This response is also neural in origin but is not cholinergic because it is blocked only by tetrodotoxin and not by atropine. Muscle strips taken from different segments of the smooth muscle portion of the esophageal body show progressively longer intervals for the off response contraction following stimulation on moving distally in the esophagus. This phenomenon has been called the latency gradient. These concepts are shown in Figure 3–7.

It has been proposed that these in vitro experiments using opossum esophagus muscle preparations may help to explain some of the mechanisms of the development of normal peristalsis in the human smooth muscle esophagus. With the initial swallowing event, an inhibitory neural discharge is sent to the circular smooth muscle of the entire esophagus. The LES relaxes from its resting tonic state. The remainder of the esophageal smooth muscle is already relaxed and shows no measurable change. Rebound contraction occurs following the end of the brief stimulus—the off response. The latency of the gradient for this off response, progressing distally down the esophagus, produces the peristaltic contraction wave. Although this concept does not entirely explain all the phenomena that have been observed in human peristaltic activity, these in vitro observations are consistent with many aspects of normal human physiology. One example is the deglutitive inhibition

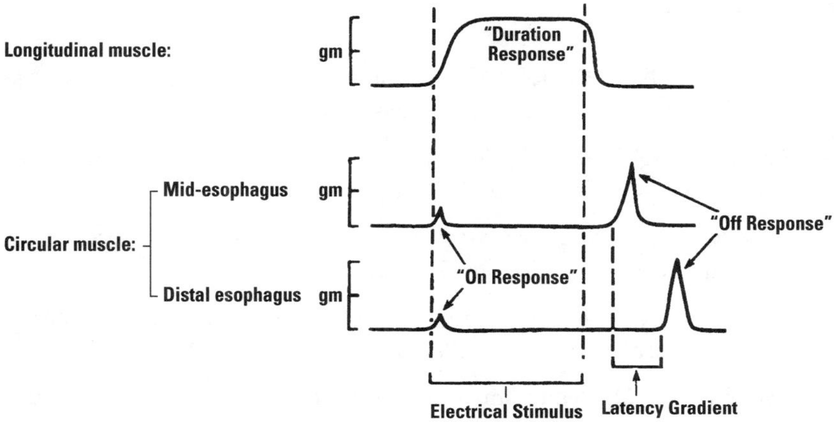

Figure 3–7. Summary of the in vitro esophageal smooth muscle responses shown in experiments in the opossum. During stimulation, the longitudinal esophageal muscle contracts throughout the stimulus; this is known as the *duration response*. The circular muscle shows a brief positive impulse at the beginning of stimulation; this is known as the *on response*. This is followed by a much greater contraction following termination of the stimulus; this is known as the *off response*. Delay in the latter response, progressing daily in the esophagus, produces the so-called latency gradient. gm = contraction force in grams.

referred to earlier. With repetitive swallowing at frequent intervals, the successive inhibitory neural impulses from the swallowing center prevent the contractions of the smooth muscle portion of the esophagus until the last swallow occurs. The off response and the latency gradient then allow the single peristaltic clearing wave that usually follows.

OTHER CONSIDERATIONS

When gastric pressure becomes greater than LES pressure, reflux occurs. It must be remembered, however, that mechanical sphincter dysfunction is not the only cause of reflux symptoms. Gastric pathology (such as hypersecretion and alkaline gastroesophageal reflux), motility disorders, and other conditions, such as impaired gastric emptying, must be considered.

REFERENCES

1. Li Q, Castell JA, Castell DO. Manometric determination of esophageal length. *Am J Gastroenterol.* 1994;89:722–725.
2. Gerhardt DC, Shuck TL, Bordeaux RA, Winship DH. Human upper esophageal sphincter. *Gastroenterology.* 1978;75:268–274.
3. Winans CS. Manometric asymmetry of the lower esophageal high pressure zone. *Am J Dig Dis.* 1977;22:348–354.
4. Meyer GW, Austin RM, Brady CE III, Castell DO. Muscle anatomy of the human esophagus. *J Clin Gastroenterol.* 1986;8:131–134.
5. Weisbrodt NW. Neuromuscular organization of esophageal and pharyngeal motility. *Arch Intern Med.* 1976;136:524–531.
6. Meyer GW, Gerhardt DC, Castell DO. Human esophageal response to rapid swallowing: muscle refractory period of neural inhibition? *Am J Physiol.* 1981;241:G129–G136.
7. Goyal RK, Rattan S. Genesis of basal sphincter pressure: effect of tetrodotoxin on the lower esophageal sphincter in opossum in vivo. *Gastroenterology.* 1976;71:62–67.
8. Richter JE, Sinar DR, Cordova CM, Castell DO. Verapamil—a potent inhibitor of esophageal contractions in the baboon. *Gastroenterology.* 1982;82:882–886.
9. Richter JE, Spurling TJ, Cordova CM, Castell DO. Effects of oral calcium blocker, diltiazem, on esophageal contractions. *Dig Dis Sci.* 1984;29:649–656.
10. Dodds WJ, Dent J, Hogan WJ, Amdorfer RJ. Effect of atropine on esophageal motor function in humans. *Am J Physiol.* 1981;240:G290–G296.
11. Pasricha PJ, Ravich WJ, Kalloo AN. Effects of intrasphincteric botulinum toxin on the lower esophageal sphincter in piglets. *Gastroenterology.* 1993;105:1045–1049.
12. Goyal RK, Rattan S, Said SI. VIP as a possible neurotransmitter of non-cholinergic non-adrenergic inhibitory neurons. *Nature.* 1980;288:378–380.
13. Sanders KM, Ward SM. Nitric oxide as a mediator of nonadrenergic noncholinergic neurotransmission. *Am J Physiol.* 1992;262:G379–G392.

14. Castell DO. The lower esophageal sphincter: physiologic and clinical aspects. *Ann Intern Med.* 1975;83:390–401.

15. Christensen J, Lund GE. Esophageal responses to distension and electrical stimulation. *J Clin Invest.* 1969;48:408–419.

4

New Concepts in the Anatomy and Physiology of the Antireflux Barrier

Larry Miller, Kian Makipour, Pathikonda Murali, and Anil Vegesna

The pathogenesis of gastroesophageal reflux disease (GERD) is complex, resulting from an imbalance between defensive factors protecting the esophagus (antireflux barriers, esophageal acid clearance, tissue resistance) and aggressive factors refluxing from the stomach (gastric acidity, volume, and duodenal contents). This chapter addresses new concepts in the anatomy and physiology of the antireflux barrier. Although there are similarities with some of the ideas discussed in Chapter 3, this chapter highlights selected new concepts that may differ from the traditional concepts reviewed in the previous chapter.

Despite extensive work, the underlying physiology and pathophysiology of the high-pressure zone (HPZ) of the distal esophagus and the underlying causes of GERD remain incompletely understood. In fact, there is still controversy regarding the anatomic components of the gastroesophageal junction (GEJ) HPZ and how these components contribute to the antireflux barrier and fail in GERD.

There are many examples in the literature where the term *lower esophageal sphincter* (LES) is used to describe the clasp and sling muscle fibers.[1,2] There are also many literature citations where "LES" is used to describe the circular smooth muscle near the distal end of the esophagus that is proximal, cephalic, or orad from the semicircular clasp and sling muscle fiber. It seems that researchers in this field have developed 2 different viewpoints. One group of researchers, primarily basic scientists, consider the LES to be the clasp and sling muscle fiber complex. Another group of researchers, primarily clinical investigators, consider the LES to be the circular smooth muscle near the distal end of the esophagus.

While the lower esophageal circular (LEC) muscle does not appear to be thicker than the more proximal esophagus in fixed autopsy specimens, it does appear thicker in vivo as observed using high resolution ultrasound. Thus, this esophageal circular smooth muscle may not have an anatomic correlate in autopsy studies. However, a series of experiments using simultaneous endoluminal ultrasound and manometry suggest that the LEC muscle complex, the semicircular gastric clasp/sling muscle fiber complex, and the crural diaphragm all exist and are important as a part of the antireflux barrier. Because of the differences in the literature concerning the exact anatomic definition of the LES, our discussion refers to specific anatomic smooth muscle fibers and uses the more specific terms *gastric sling muscle fibers, gastric clasp muscle fibers,* and *LEC muscle fibers* for these structures. When these could not be reconciled in the literature, the term "LES" is used. Unfortunately, it is not always possible in the historical literature to distinguish among these structures, and it is not possible in most circumstances to determine to which structure the authors are referring.

COMPONENTS OF THE GASTROESOPHAGEAL JUNCTION HIGH-PRESSURE ZONE

We introduce the concept of a 3-component HPZ in the area of the GEJ. The sphincteric components within the GEJ regulate the flow of food from the esophagus into the stomach; allow venting of gas and regurgitation from the stomach; and act as an antireflux barrier to gastric content. Several muscle groups are important in maintaining an antireflux barrier. The intrinsic muscles of the distal 4 cm of the esophagus (LEC muscle) and proximal stomach (gastric clasp/sling muscle fiber complex) constitute the internal, smooth muscle mechanism of the HPZ. The crural diaphragm, positioned between and overlapping these, constitutes the external, skeletal muscle mechanism. The phrenoesophageal ligament anchors the distal esophagus to the crural diaphragm.[3] Since the LEC smooth muscle component, the crural diaphragm, and the gastric clasp/sling muscle fiber complex are anatomically contiguous in normal individuals, intraluminal pressure is due to the combination of all of these muscles. Distinguishing the individual components reveals the contribution of each structure to the antireflux barrier and identifies which components are defective in GERD.

Lower Esophageal Circular Muscle

The circular muscles of the most distal 2 to 3 cm of the lower esophagus are thicker than those of the adjacent esophagus, as previously described.[4] Muscle thickness is directly related to sphincter contraction and pressure; the muscle becomes thinner with stretching and thicker with shortening during respiration, swallowing, and compression by the crural diaphragm.[5] The rich nerve supply of the LEC differs from the remainder of the tubular esophagus. The myenteric plexus lies in several muscle planes of the LEC, whereas in the body of the esophagus, the plexus lies between the longitudinal and circular muscle layers.

Crural Diaphragm

The diaphragm is composed of costal and crural components, which are attached to the vertebral column. These 2 diaphragmatic components have separate embryologic origins and different functions. The costal diaphragm is involved in respiratory activity, whereas the crural diaphragm is not. The crural diaphragm forms a canal through which the esophagus enters the abdomen. Contraction of the crural diaphragm exerts a pinchcock-like action at the GEJ HPZ, thereby forming an extrinsic sphincter mechanism.[3] The diaphragmatic component of the HPZ can be isolated from the esophageal components with the use of cisatracurium, which paralyzes the skeletal muscle of the crural diaphragm but not the smooth muscle, as demonstrated in our prior studies.[6] The crural diaphragm alone can maintain a zone of high-pressure at the abdominal thoracic junction in patients who have undergone esophagogastrectomy, as shown by Drs Parkman and Fisher.[7] Our group quantitated the contribution of the crural diaphragm in normal volunteers and in patients with GERD and demonstrated an anatomic asymmetry of the crural diaphragm in normal control subjects.[8]

GASTRIC CLASP/SLING MUSCLE FIBER PRESSURE PROFILE

The arrangement of the smooth muscle fibers at the GEJ has been described based on an anatomic study of 32 cadavers.[9] The musculature consists of clasp muscle fibers on the lesser curvature side and sling muscle fibers on the greater curvature side of the cardia of the stomach. The gastric clasp/sling muscle fiber complex acts as the first barrier to reflux of gastric contents. In GERD patients, the contribution of the gastric clasp/sling muscle fiber complex to the GEJ pressure profile is absent.[8]

Until now, it has not been possible to accurately separate the GEJ HPZ into its component parts and to study the mechanical properties of these components individually. We were able to accomplish this in normal volunteers and in GERD patients using a technique that employs ultrasonography and manometry simultaneously during pharmacologic manipulation of the GEJ HPZ. The smooth muscle components consisting of the LEC muscle fibers and the gastric clasp/sling muscle fiber complex were inhibited by the muscarinic antagonist atropine. In a separate study, the skeletal muscle component (crural diaphragm) was paralyzed with the nicotinic receptor antagonist and neuromuscular blocking agent cisatracurium.

ANATOMY AND PHYSIOLOGY OF THE GEJ HPZ IN NORMAL CONTROL SUBJECTS

In early studies, our group developed the technique of simultaneous endoluminal ultrasound and manometry to evaluate the HPZ of the distal esophagus and differentiate the pressure profile generated by the intrinsic smooth muscle fibers from the pressure profile generated by the external skeletal muscle of the crural diaphragm.[10] We then identified the anatomic and physiologic relationships among the 3 components of the GEJ HPZ: the LEC muscle fibers, the crural diaphragm, and the gastric clasp/sling muscle fiber complex. This was done in 15 healthy volunteers during breath holding of inspiration and expiration. Pressure was determined during pull-through of the catheter assembly at a constant velocity before and after intravenous administration of the muscarinic receptor antagonist atropine.[6] The average difference between the pre-atropine and post-atropine pressure profiles for these 15 volunteers is shown in blue in Figure 4–1. Two distinct peaks are seen in both inspiration and expiration, roughly 1.5 to 1.6 cm apart. The distal peaks on the left of each graph represent the gastric clasp/sling muscle fiber pressure profile, while the proximal peaks on the right represent the pressure exerted by the LEC muscle fibers.

The findings were further confirmed with the neuromuscular blocking agent cisatracurium in 7 patients undergoing general anesthesia

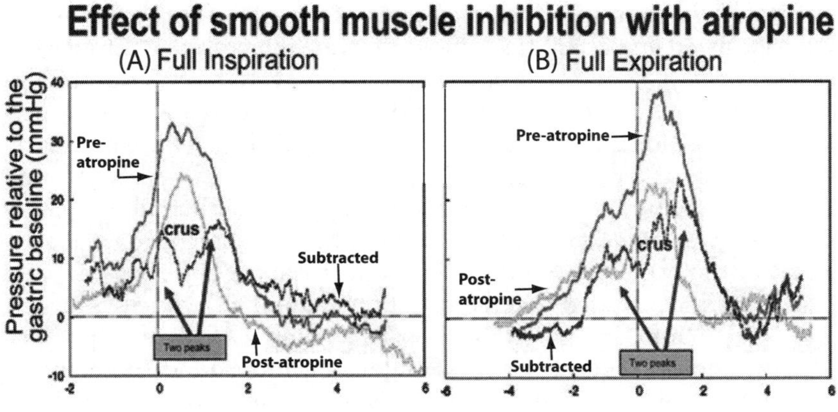

Figure 4–1. Averaged pressure distributions from pull-throughs referenced to the lower margin of the crus muscles with the costal diaphragm (RCd). Full inspiration (A); full expiration (B). The continuous curves are obtained by subtracting the post-atropine pressure distribution from the complete pressure distribution, for each pull-through, giving the contribution to tone that is sensitive to atropine. The dashed curves are the atropine-resistant pressure distributions, and the thin dotted lines are the baseline pressure distributions reflecting the summation of all sphincteric components.

for non-esophageal surgery.[10] Once again, the same 2 peaks, in the same anatomic location with respect to the crural diaphragm, were seen after skeletal muscle paralysis. Thus, 2 different pharmacologic agents provided the same findings that distinguished the 2 smooth muscle components of the GEJ HPZ from the skeletal muscle component (the crural diaphragm): the LEC muscle fibers overlap the crural diaphragm and are located proximal to the crural diaphragm, and the gastric clasp/sling muscle fiber complex overlaps the crural diaphragm and is located distal to this skeletal muscle component.

THE NORMAL OVERLAPPING GASTROESOPHAGEAL SPHINCTERS

Several recent studies[4,6,10] used simultaneous ultrasound and manometry to study the anatomy and physiology of the GEJ HPZ. High-frequency ultrasound was co-localized with manometric pressure during breath holding under full inspiration and full expiration with a machine pull-through of a simultaneous ultrasound/manometry catheter assembly from the stomach into the thoracic esophagus. For each pull-through, axial locations of the margins of the right crus muscle were localized and quantified. Pressures were referenced to intragastric pressure. Spatial references used in this study were the inferior margin of the right crus of the diaphragm and the initiation of the pull-through (its start position). The in vivo results showed that the mean muscle thickness in the region of the GEJ HPZ increases continuously through the abdominal esophagus to the esophagocardiac junction. Muscle thickness was highly nonuniform around the lumen perimeter; at each axial location, the maximum/minimum thickness ratio was at least 150%. It was concluded that the variation in muscle thickness is largest where the diaphragmatic crus contacts the outer wall of the esophagus. McCray and colleagues,[10] using simultaneous ultrasound and manometry, noted that the crural diaphragm was anatomically superimposed on the intrinsic LEC proximal to the GEJ, causing compression so that the anatomy of the sphincter within the distal esophagus appears asymmetric, thus accounting for the asymmetry in the pressure profile.

Brasseur and colleagues[6] used simultaneous ultrasound and manometry to study the gastroesophageal HPZ with pharmacologic manipulation, evaluating the anatomic and physiologic relationships among the various components of the GEJ HPZ. Using this technique, it was possible to evaluate how each component of the GEJ HPZ moved with respect to each of the other components during respiration. It was found that the crus muscle moved ~1.9 cm between inspiration and expiration. The inferior margin of the right crus muscle was found to be at the inferior margin of the post-atropine HPZ in both full inspiration and full expiration. The anatomic crus was 2 cm in length, independent of positioning of the costal diaphragm, indicating that the axial length of the crural diaphragm remains constant during respiration. The upper intrinsic sphincter moved rigidly with the crural diaphragm, indicating a tight attachment with the phrenoesophageal ligament. The upper intrinsic sphincter and crural sphincter separated by about 1 cm from the lower intrinsic sphincter (gastric clasp/sling muscle fiber complex) during inferior-to-superior excursion of the costal diaphragm.

In summary, Brasseur et al[6] concluded that the HPZ of the distal esophagus is composed of 3 components. The 2 intrinsic components are: (1) an upper physiologic sphincter (the LEC muscle) that overlaps and moves with the crural sphincter and (2) a lower anatomic component at the junction between the gastric cardia and esophagus, formed by the gastric clasp/sling muscle fiber complex. The extrinsic component, the crural diaphragm, is attached to the LEC muscle by the phrenoesophageal ligament and moves in lockstep with the LEC during respiration, separating from the gastric clasp/sling muscle fiber complex during expiration.

ANATOMY AND PHYSIOLOGY OF THE GEJ HPZ IN GERD PATIENTS

A comparable study to that of Brasseur et al[6] was performed in 7 GERD patients.[11] The subtraction curve in Figure 4–2 demonstrates that the distal peak pressure profile due to the gastric clasp/sling muscle fiber complex is absent. The proximal peak representing the LEC fibers was present in the same axial location relative to the crural diaphragm as in the normal volunteers.

Miller et al,[8] using simultaneous ultrasound and manometry, discovered that an abnormality of the gastric clasp/sling muscle fiber complex exists in patients who have GERD. The distal pressure profile caused by the gastric clasp/sling muscle fiber complex, seen in normal control subjects, was lacking in patients who had GERD (Figure 4–3). The relative contributions of each of the components of the GEJ HPZ were evaluated and compared in GERD patients and normal control subjects, to determine which abnormalities predispose patients to reflux. High-frequency endoluminal ultrasound and simultaneous manometry were used to evaluate patients who had GERD during inspiration and

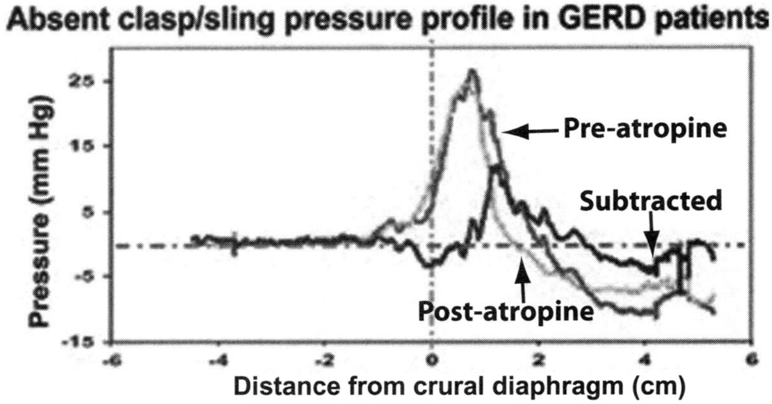

Figure 4–2. Average from 7 patients with GERD. Pre-atropine, post-atropine, and subtracted—pre-atropine minus post-atropine—curves are indicated. Note that the distal peak from the gastric clasp/sling muscle fiber complex is completely absent.

expiration, as in the previous studies in normal volunteers. Earlier, the normal intrinsic sphincter HPZ was described as containing 2 peaks that separate between inspiration and expiration. However, in all GERD patients, the intrinsic sphincter pressure profiles displayed a complete absence of the distal peak in both inspiration and expiration, indicating an absence of tone in the gastric clasp/sling muscle fiber complex. The proximal pressure peak, reflecting the physiologic LEC muscle in the abdominal esophagus, was present in the same axial location relative to the crural diaphragm as in the normal volunteers. It was concluded that GERD patients lack the pressure profile consistent with the gastric clasp/sling muscle fiber complex.

INDUCED LOWER ESOPHAGEAL SPHINCTER RELAXATION

Many patients with GERD have normal resting LES pressure on manometry, suggesting that other factors must contribute to the pathogenesis of GERD. A static measurement of pressure, using conventional techniques, is not a true assessment of LES function. LES pressure may be abnormally low on a transient rather than a sustained basis. The mechanism of GERD is most commonly attributed to transient LES relaxations,[12–15] which are prolonged relaxations of the GEJ HPZ, occur-

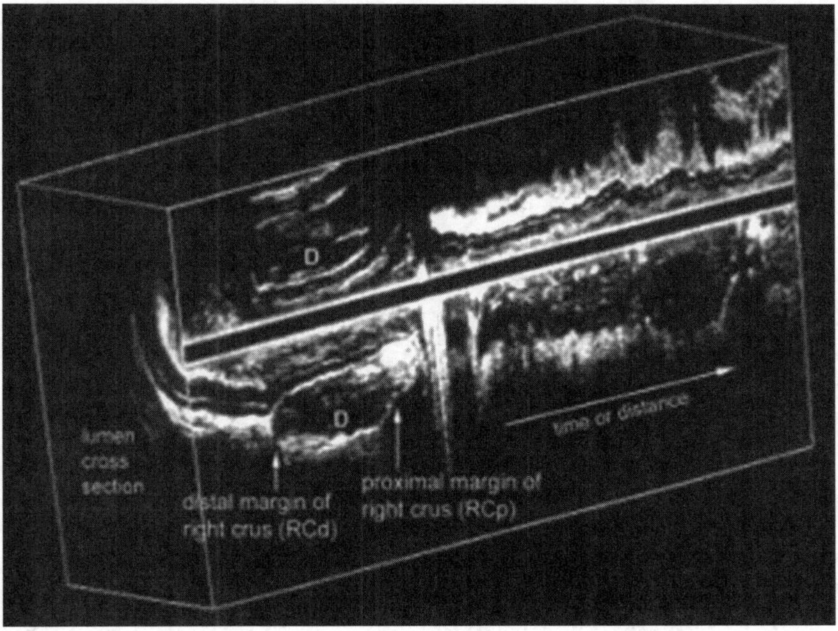

Figure 4–3. Three-dimensional reconstruction of ultrasound images from a pull-through of the distal oesophagus and surrounding structures The images are stacked in time where the left-most portion of the image is the abdominal oesophagus and the right-most portion is the mediastinum. Half the oesophagus is sliced away with the catheter in the centre. The left-most cross-section shows the circular and longitudinal layers of the muscularis propria separated by connective tissue. The hypoechoic area outside the lumen of the oesophagus is the crural diaphragm, labelled with a "D." The margin of the right crus distal (RCd) and margin of the right crus proximal (RCp) are indicated.

ring spontaneously, in the absence of swallowing. The cardiac region of the stomach has the lowest threshold for triggering stretch-induced LES relaxation.[16–19] This is exactly the area where distensibility is increased in GERD patients, presumably due to the abnormal gastric clasp/sling muscle fiber complex.[8,18,19,20]

Vagal cooling abolishes the triggering of gastric cardia stretch-induced LES relaxation,[21] suggesting mediation by a vagal reflex. Gastric cardia stretch-induced LES relaxations are integrated motor responses, which involve crural diaphragm inhibition.[21] Transient LES relaxations are difficult to study because they are infrequent, isolated events. We developed a method to induce LES relaxation in order to trigger the transient kind at will. This was accomplished by distending the stomach with air during endoscopy and determining the intragastric pressure and volume threshold required for inducing LES relaxation in normal control subjects and in GERD patients without hiatal hernia.[22]

Thirteen normal volunteers and 3 patients with GERD underwent endoscopy. A pressure transducer was placed through the biopsy channel of the endoscope. Air was removed from the stomach with the endoscope in a retroflexed position, and a gastric baseline pressure was measured. Air was then insufflated into the stomach through the endoscope at a constant flow until the GEJ opened or until the subject complained of discomfort. The volume of air and the pressure above the baseline were measured at the time of GEJ opening on the endoscopic view. This was repeated 3 to 4 times in each subject, and the results of these repeated trials were averaged. In the 13 normal volunteers, the mean pressure and volume of GEJ opening was 12 ± 9 mm Hg and 1284 ± 570 mL, respectively. In the 3 GERD patients, the average GEJ opening pressure and volume were 3 ± 5 mm Hg and 221 ± 452 mL, significantly lower than in the normal control subjects ($p < .001$).[22]

The photograph on the left in Figure 4–4 shows a retroflexed view of the GEJ in a normal volunteer. The white catheter is the manometry catheter, and the black tube is the endoscope. Note that the GEJ

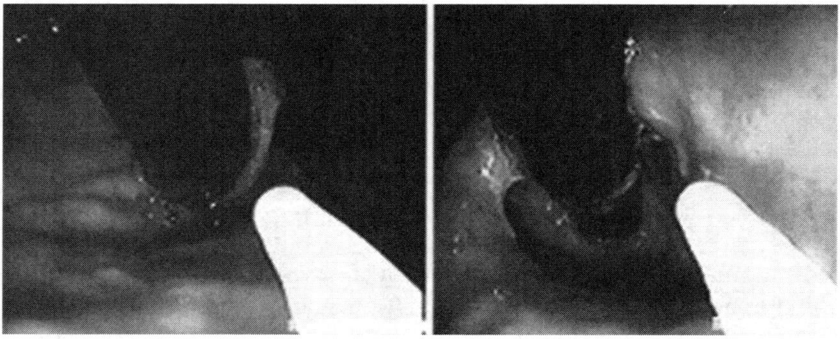

Figure 4–4. This is pattern II opening. This picture shows a retroflexed view of the gastroesophageal junction in a normal volunteer. The white catheter is the manometry catheter and the black tube is the endoscope. Note that the hiatus is open around the endoscope during air insufflation into the stomach but that the distal esophagus remains closed and tight around the endoscope. This subject did not have a hiatal hernia, and the esophagus was tight around the endoscope prior to air insufflation.

is tight around the endoscope prior to air insufflation into the stomach. The photograph on the right in Figure 4–4 shows a view of the same subject after air insufflation into the stomach. Note that the GEJ is open around the endoscope, yet the more proximal portion of the GEJ HPZ is still tightly closed around the endoscope. This portion of the GEJ HPZ opened at a higher intragastric pressure and volume than the distal portion of the GEJ HPZ. Subsequent studies using stationary high-resolution manometry catheters across the GEJ HPZ demonstrated the same phenomenon, confirming the sequential relaxation of the individual components of the GEJ HPZ.

HIATAL HERNIA

Hiatal hernia is implicated in the pathogenesis of GERD[17,23] and is frequently encountered in patients with GERD. However, not all patients with hiatal hernia have symptoms of GERD. Normally, the LES is reinforced by the diaphragm to form an HPZ preventing reflux of gastric contents into the esophagus.[24] This reflux-preventing mechanism is disrupted when the LES is displaced into the chest along with part of the stomach, allowing reflux. Food and gastric secretions can also be trapped in the hiatal hernia sac to reflux proximally, especially when it undergoes fermentation. Surgical correction of the hiatal hernia with lengthening of the esophagus and closure of the diaphragmatic crura can restore the HPZ. Vigorous exercise or lifting weights can disrupt the repair, leading to recurrence of symptoms.

ROLE OF THE MUCOSA IN PREVENTING GERD

There are 4 main fundamental factors that are considered important in the development of GERD: (1) gastric acid; (2) the structural integrity, function, and competence of the HPZ of the distal esophagus that either prevents or allows reflux; (3) the esophageal mucosal defense mechanisms that are primarily called into play when there is excess exposure of the mucosa to gastric acid; and (4) the sensory mechanisms that speak to symptoms. That is, an incompetent GERD mechanism allows abnormal amounts of gastric acid to enter the esophagus, where the acid burden causes mucosal damage and/or symptoms.

The mucosa of the esophagus plays a major role in protecting the underlying muscle layer. It is the first line of defense for the lower esophagus against the acid from the stomach. The major mucosal defenses against acid of the squamous mucosa of the esophagus are by luminal acid clearance and tissue resistance. Tissue resistance has 3 defense components: the pre-epithelial, the epithelial, and the post-epithelial. The pre-epithelial defense consists of surface mucus and an unstirred water layer within which bicarbonate ions are trapped, providing an alkaline microenvironment. The epithelial defense consists of the apical cell membranes and junctional complexes, which act to limit the diffusion of H^+ from lumen to cell and intercellular space, respectively. The post-epithelial defense is provided by the acid-buffering effects of HCO_3- in cells and within the intracellular space. Blood supply is essential for the delivery of HCO_3-.

In previous in vivo studies in human subjects, we observed some very interesting and unique phenomena regarding the esophagus during deglutition. In one study, using simultaneous endoluminal ultrasound and manometry in the distal esophagus at the level of the distal HPZ, we observed that during deglutition, the mucosa in the distal esophagus shortened coincident with the relaxation of the HPZ and that the gastric mucosa was actually pulled up into the distal portion of the esophagus during swallowing.[25]

In yet another study, using transabdominal ultrasound during deglutition, we observed that the mucosa of the distal esophagus shortened well before the rest of the esophagus did so and that the mucosa, by shortening proximally and pulling up the gastric mucosa, formed a narrow channel in the distal esophageal lumen through which fluid shot through in a proximal to distal direction.[26]

Preliminary studies demonstrate that in patients with GERD, the mucosa does not shorten during swallowing. This may be an effect of the reflux or it may represent a primary pathophysiology in the development of GERD.[25] We believe, based on the results of these studies, that the muscularis mucosa of the distal esophagus may participate in the protection of the distal esophagus through a unique mechanism. The mucosa may act as an antireflux mechanism by forming a partial plug or one-way valve during deglutition. Theoretically, this would act to protect the esophagus from reflux of gastric contents between the time that the HPZ relaxes at the initiation of swallowing and the time that the bolus reaches the distal esophagus. It is during this period of time that there is no effective protective pressure barrier. If the intra-abdominal pressure should be greater than the intrathoracic pressure, the pressure differential would lead to fluid flow from the stomach into the esophagus.[25,26]

In summary, the underlying physiology and pathophysiology of the HPZ of the distal esophagus and the underlying causes of GERD remain incompletely understood. In this chapter we introduced the concept of the 3-component HPZ antireflux barrier in the distal esophagus and proximal stomach. We demonstrated that these 3 components consist of the LEC muscle in the distal esophagus, the crural diaphragm (extrinsinc skeletal muscle component), and the gastric clasp/sling muscle fiber complex in the proximal stomach. We showed that the traditional view of a static sphincter is incorrect and that each of the individual components moves and changes tone with respect to the other components during inspiration and expiration. We demonstrated that in GERD patients, the pressure profile due to the gastric clasp/sling muscle fiber components are defective. Furthermore, this defect in the tone of the clasp/sling muscle fiber components appears to allow increased distensibility of the cardia of the stomach and therefore may allow initiation of transient LES relaxations (a vagally mediated reflex) at a lower threshold than in normal individuals. Finally, we demonstrated that during swallowing, the muscularis mucosa of the esophagus causes the gastric mucosa to be pulled up from the cardia into the distal esophagus. This leads to the formation of a narrow channel in the distal esophageal lumen through which fluid jets through in a proximal-to-distal direction. Thus, the mucosa may act as an antireflux mechanism by forming a partial plug or one-way valve during deglutition. This occurs during a period of time that the rest of the HPZ is relaxed (all 3 components of the HPZ relax upon the initiation of deglutition). Therefore, this mechanism may prevent reflux at a point in time when the gastric pressure is higher than the thoracic pressure and there is no other antireflux barrier. Preliminary studies demonstrate that in patients with GERD, the mucosa does not shorten during swallowing.

REFERENCES

1. Farre R, Auli M, Lecea B, Martinez E, Clave P. Pharmacologic characterization of intrinsic mechanisms controlling tone and relaxation of porcine lower esophageal sphincter. *J Pharmacol Experimental Ther.* 2006;316:1238–1248.
2. Gonzalez AA, Farre R, Clave P. Different responsiveness of excitatory and inhibitory enteric motor neurons in the human esophagus to electrical field stimulation and to nicotine. *Am J Physiol Gastrointest Liver Physiol.* 2004;287:G299–G306.
3. Boyle JT, Altschuler SM, Nixon TE, Tuchman DN, Pack AI, Cohen S. Role of the diaphragm in the genesis of lower esophageal sphincter pressure in the cat. *Surv Anesthesiol.* 1985;29:319.

4. Liu JB, Miller LS, Goldberg BB, Feld RI, Alexander AA, Needleman L, Castell DO, Klenn PJ, Millward CL. Transnasal US of the esophagus: preliminary morphologic and function studies. *Radiology*. 1992;184:721–727.

5. Liu J, Parashar VK, Mittal RK. Asymmetry of lower esophageal sphincter pressure: is it related to the muscle thickness or its shape? *Am J Physiol Gastrointest Liver Physiol*. 1997;272:G1509–G1517.

6. Brasseur JG, Ulerich R, Dai Q, Patel DK, Soliman AMS, Miller LS. Pharmacological dissection of the human gastro-oesophageal segment into three sphincteric components. *J Physiol*. 2007;580:961–975.

7. Klein WA, Parkman HP, Dempsey DT, Fisher RS. Sphincterlike thoracoabdominal high pressure zone after esophagogastrectomy. *Gastroenterology*. 1993;105:1362–1369.

8. Miller L, Dai Q, Vegesna A, et al. A missing sphincteric component of the gastro-oesophageal junction in patients with GORD. *Neurogastroenterol Motil*. 2009;21:813–e52.

9. Liebermann-Meffert D, Allgower M, Schmid P, Blum AL. Muscular equivalent of the lower esophageal sphincter. *Gastroenterology*. 1979; 76:31–38.

10. McCray WH, Chung C, Parkman HP, Miller LS. Use of simultaneous high-resolution endoluminal sonography (HRES) and manometry to characterize high pressure zone of distal esophagus. *Dig Dis Sci*. 2000;45:1660–1666.

11. Miller LS, Brasseur J, Ulerich R, Thomas B, Thomas A, Dai Q. A new theory to explain the pathophysiology of GERD. Pharmacological separation of the gastro-esophageal junction high pressure zone (GEJHPZ) demonstrates an absent gastric sling fiber pressure profile in patients with GERD. *Gastroenterology*. 2004;126:T1741.

12. Hornby PJ, Abrahams TP. Central control of lower esophageal sphincter relaxation. *Am J Med*. 2000;108:90–98.

13. Mittal RK, Holloway R, Dent J. Effect of atropine on the frequency of reflux and transient lower esophageal sphincter relaxation in normal subjects. *Gastroenterology*. 1995;109:1547–1554.

14. Dent J, Dodds WJ, Friedman RH, et al. Mechanism of gastroesophageal reflux in recumbent asymptomatic human subjects. *J Clin Invest*. 1980;65:256–267.

15. Dodds WJ, Dent J, Hogan WJ, Arndorfer RC. Effect of atropine on esophageal motor function in humans. *Am J Physiol Gastrointest Liver Physiol.* 1981;240:G290–G296.

16. Franzi SJ, Martin CJ, Cox MR, Dent J. Response of canine lower esophageal sphincter to gastric distension. *Am J Physiol Gastrointest Liver Physiol.* 1990;259:G380–G385.

17. Kahrilas PJ, Shi G, Manka M, Joehl RJ. Increased frequency of transient lower esophageal sphincter relaxation induced by gastric distention in reflux patients with hiatal hernia. *Gastroenterology.* 2000;118:688–695.

18. Holloway HR, Hongo M, Berger K, McCallum WR. *Gastric Distention: A Mechanism for Postprandial Gastroesophageal Reflux.* New York, NY: Wiley; 1985.

19. Straathof JWA, van Veen MM, Masclee AAM. Provocation of transient lower esophageal sphincter relaxations during continuous gastric distension. *Scand J Gastroenterol.* 2002;37:1140–1143.

20. Schiffner BJ, Miller L, Dai Q, Dimitriou J, Brasseur JG. Opening stiffness and geometry of the esophago-gastric segment in health, with GERD, and after endoscopic surgery. *Gastroenterology.* 2005;128: M1808, A397–A398.

21. Martin JC, Patrikios J, Dent J. *Abolition of Gas Reflux and Transient Lower Esophagea Sphincter Relaxation by Vagal Blockade in the Dog.* New York, NY: Wiley; 1986.

22. Vegesna A, Besetty R, Kalra A, et al. Induced opening of the gastroesophageal junction occurs at a lower gastric pressure in GERD patients and in hiatal hernia subjects than in normal control subjects. *Gastroenterol Res Pract.* 2010.

23. Kahrilas PJ. Anatomy and physiology of the gastroesophageal junction. *Gastroenterol Clin North Am.* 1997;26:467–486.

24. Miller L, Vegesna A, Kalra A, et al. New observations on the gastroesophageal antireflux barrier. *Gastroenterol Clin North Am.* 2007;36: 601–617.

25. Hussain K, Bilal F, Patel H, et al. Assessment of mucosal movement in the gastroesophageal junction high-pressure zone during swallowing using simultaneous endoluminal ultrasound and manometry. *Gastroenterology.* 2011;140:S-471.

26. Vegesna AK, Indukuri S, Nimma A, Bhatti H, Makipour K, Miller LS. Evaluation of the gastroesophageal junction high pressure zone using transabdominal ultrasound during bolus transit. *Gastroenterology*. 2011;140:S-620.

5

Gastroesophageal Reflux Disease: An Overview of Clinical Presentation and Epidemiology

Gastroesophageal reflux disease (GERD) is a spectrum of disease best defined as symptoms and/or signs of esophageal or adjacent organ injury that are secondary to the reflux of gastric contents into the esophagus or above into the oral cavity or airways. GERD is a common disorder, often encountered in clinical practice, and patients present with a multitude of symptoms. Injury caused by GERD is defined on the basis of the location of symptoms or organ damage, which includes esophagitis; inflammation of the larynx, pharynx, and oral cavity; and acute and/or chronic pulmonary injury. This chapter presents an overview of GERD, including typical, atypical, and extraesophageal presentations.

TYPICAL SYMPTOMS

The typical or classic symptoms of GERD are heartburn, or pyrosis (burning occurring shortly after meals or on bending over and relieved with antacids), and regurgitation (the spontaneous return of gastric contents into the esophagus or mouth). When present together, heartburn and regurgitation establish a clinical diagnosis with a high degree of confidence, and a trial of medical therapy can be instituted. In clinical practice, heartburn is a daily complaint in 7% to 10% of the population in the United States, and at least monthly in ~40% to 50%.[1–3] More than 20 million Americans have heartburn at least twice a week and use antacids or other over-the-counter antireflux products on a regular basis. Troublesome regurgitation is experienced by ~16% of the population, according to one study.[2] The frequency of heartburn probably does not change—however, the intensity of symptoms appears to decrease slightly with increasing age. There does not appear to be a gender difference in GERD symptoms, though erosive esophagitis is more frequent in men, as is Barrett's esophagus and adenocarcinoma. Symptoms are likely equal in frequency in the United States in Caucasians and African Americans. GERD symptoms are more common in obese patients, who are at greater risk for Barrett's esophagus and adenocarcinoma.

Classic heartburn is described typically by patients as a burning sensation under the breastbone radiating upward toward the throat or mouth. Heartburn generally occurs 1 to 2 hours after meals, following heavy lifting, or on bending over. Big meals, spicy foods, citrus products such as grapefruit and orange juice, and meals high in fat are most likely to produce heartburn. Cola drinks, coffee, teas, and even beer may have an acidic pH and cause symptoms when ingested. Heartburn may also be caused by medications (Table 5–1). Eating meals late in the evening, close to bedtime, or with alcohol makes patients more prone to night-

Table 5-1. Factors Causing Exacerbation of Heartburn

Decreases LES Pressure	Mucosal Irritant
Food and beverages	Food and beverages
Fats	Citrus products
Chocolate	Tomato products
Onions	Spicy foods
Carminatives	Coffee, cola drinks, tea, beer
Coffee	
Alcohol	Medications
Smoking	Aspirin
Medications	NSAIDs
Progesterone	Tetracycline
Theophylline	Quinidine
Anticholinergic agents	Progesterone
β-Adrenergic agonists	Potassium tablets
α-Adrenergic antagonists	Iron salts
Diazepam	Alendronate
Meperidine	Zidovudine
Nitrates	
Calcium channel-blockers	

LES = lower esophageal sphincter; NSAIDs = nonsteroidal anti-inflammatory drugs.

time symptoms. Patients report often that their symptoms are relieved by an over-the-counter antacid preparation or histamine-2 receptor antagonists, or even by drinking water.

Although heartburn is often associated with regurgitation, in which the patient spontaneously experiences an acidic or bitter taste in the throat or mouth, they are not synonymous symptoms. Heartburn should not be confused with dyspepsia, that is, a more vague epigastric distress usually localized to the upper abdominal or lower substernal area and associated with nausea, bloating, or a sensation of fullness after meals. Although dyspepsia (epigastric discomfort) may be a symptom of GERD, it is neither as sensitive nor as specific a symptom as heartburn. The generic term "acid indigestion" used to encompass all symptoms related to GERD is inappropriate; specific symptoms must be identified for accurate diagnosis and therapy. Water brash, the sudden filling of the mouth with a clear, salty fluid, should not be confused with heartburn. This symptom reflects the increase in salivary secretion occurring as a reflex response to reflux or to regurgitation of gastric acid into an inflamed distal esophagus.

Heartburn is a highly specific symptom of GERD, although GERD is not the only cause. For example, a heartburn-like symptom, suspected to be due to esophageal stasis from outflow obstruction, is described often in patients with achalasia. It is thought that fermentation of undigested food in the esophagus coupled with inflammation may create a heartburn-like sensation in the absence of true GERD. Functional heartburn may also be a component of irritable bowel syndrome. However, if heartburn is the only presenting esophageal symptom, it is probably due to GERD.

Despite the sensitivity and specificity of these 2 symptoms for the diagnosis of GERD, neither the presence of heartburn and/or regurgitation nor the frequency of these symptoms is predictive of the degree of damage to the distal esophagus as seen on endoscopy. Many patients with daily heartburn have no endoscopic abnormalities. The frequency of heartburn usually does not correlate with the severity of GERD, although nocturnal heartburn suggests the possibility of erosive esophagitis. Only 50% to 60% of patients presenting with heartburn will have erosive esophagitis seen on a diagnostic endoscopic examination; the remainder will be diagnosed as having nonerosive GERD.[4] Patients with severe disease, including Barrett's esophagus and peptic strictures, may present with infrequent or absent complaints of heartburn.

In most patients with esophagitis, the disease does not progress beyond the severity seen at the time of initial endoscopy. In a series of 701 patients evaluated over follow-up periods ≤29 years, progression to a more serious grade of esophagitis was seen in only 23%.[5] The patient with reflux symptoms and no evidence of esophagitis (nonerosive GERD) has even less likelihood of esophageal disease progression to a higher grade, seen over 6 months in <15% of patients.[6]

Regurgitation is often associated with heartburn and GERD. When the 2 symptoms are present together, the diagnosis of GERD is highly likely. Regurgitation without heartburn should raise suspicion of Barrett's esophagus (in which acid sensitivity is reduced), achalasia, or other esophageal abnormality. Regurgitation may also be a more prominent symptom in extraesophageal presentations of GERD, particularly in patients with pulmonary symptoms of reflux, and it may be an important prognostic factor in predicting outcome of therapy.[7,8] Regurgitation is often perceived by patients as vomiting, but the former is characterized by the effortless return of food or fluid in the absence of nausea—an important distinction to make. Esophageal and extraesophageal symptoms associated with GERD are outlined in Table 5–2.

Table 5-2. Symptoms Associated with Gastroesophageal Reflux

Esophageal	Extraesophageal
Chest pain	Asthma or respiratory problems (ie, wheezing or shortnesss of breath)
Dysphagia	Chronic cough
Heartburn	Dental hypersensitivity (from loss of dental enamel)
Odynophagia (rare)	Laryngitis or laryngospasm
Regurgitation	Nausea
Water brash	Otalgia

EXTRAESOPHAGEAL (ATYPICAL) SYMPTOMS

A number of so-called atypical or extraesophageal symptoms have been associated with GERD, including unexplained substernal chest pain without evidence of coronary artery disease (noncardiac chest pain), asthma, bronchitis, chronic cough, recurrent pneumonia, hoarseness, chronic posterior laryngitis, globus sensation, otalgia, aphthous ulcers, hiccups, and erosion of dental enamel. In contrast to heartburn and regurgitation, the prevalence of these atypical or extraesophageal symptoms and their frequency in the general population have not been systematically studied until fairly recently. In a large population-based survey of whites in Olmsted County, Minnesota,[2] designed to assess the prevalence of GERD in the general population, unexplained chest pain was reported by 23% of the population yearly and by 4% at least weekly. Surprisingly, the frequency of unexplained chest pain decreased with age. Forty percent had symptoms >5 years, and 5% reported severe symptoms. Asthma was reported in ~9%, bronchitis in ~20%, and chronic cough in 15% of patients who had atypical GERD symptoms.

The association of these atypical symptoms with heartburn and regurgitation is controversial. In the Minnesota study, 2 patients with heartburn and regurgitation had 1 or more atypical symptoms ~80% of the time. Atypical symptoms were more common in patients with frequent GERD symptoms than in patients with no GERD symptoms. Heartburn or regurgitation was reported in >80% of the patients with unexplained chest pain and in 60% with globus sensation. The only exception was asthma: ~60% of patients with asthma, bronchitis, hoarseness, and pneumonia had heartburn or regurgitation. The presence of heartburn is not predictive of otolaryngologic symptoms. However, in a case control study by the Veterans Administration,[9] patients with a discharge diagnosis of erosive esophagitis had twice the prevalence of an associated otolaryngologic symptom noted in control patients without esophagitis. Observations in patients presenting with atypical GERD show that frequent heartburn and regurgitation are uncommon complaints; however, the absence of these typical symptoms should not preclude making a diagnosis. Prospective studies using endoscopy and ambulatory pH monitoring find GERD in as many as 75% of patients with chronic hoarseness,[10] in 70% to 80% of asthmatics,[11,12] and in 20% of patients with chronic cough.[13]

Reflux is a well-recognized cause of atypical chest pain and may be responsible for many (or most) of the symptoms in 75,000 to 150,000 patients who undergo normal coronary angiography in the United States annually.[14]

Approximately 45% of patients with unexplained chest pain can be shown to have GERD.[15] Esophagitis in this population is less common, being seen in <10%.[16] Endoscopically, esophagitis is seen in 30% to 40% of patients with asthma[17,18] and ~20% of patients with reflux laryngitis. Distinguishing between cardiac and noncardiac chest pain due to GERD is difficult, and they may coexist in the same patient. All the features of cardiac angina—tight, gripping, viselike pain radiating to the neck, shoulder, or left arm and associated with exertion—may be seen with GERD also. Prolonged pain (lasting >1 h), pain relieved by eating, or pain on awakening from sleep is more likely to be of esophageal origin. Antacids or histamine-2 blockers may relieve chest pain that is later proved to be associated with coronary artery disease. It is therefore crucial to rule out cardiac disease before GERD is presumed to be the cause of chest pain. Omeprazole therapy is effective for reflux-related noncardiac chest pain[19]; and in patients with frequent (<3 times/wk), noncardiac chest pain, high-dose proton-pump inhibitor (PPI) therapy may be a sensitive, specific, cost-effective strategy for diagnosing GERD.[20] However, it must be remembered that not all patients respond to PPI medications. Therefore, the persistence of chest pain during PPI therapy does not definitively rule out GERD as the cause of the chest pain, as the evaluation of patients with unexplained chest pain remains complex.[21]

For example, the rare syndrome X is a condition involving angina chest pain with objective signs of ischemia on exercise stress testing or myocardial scintigraphy, but with normal coronary arteries on angiogram. Esophageal hypersensitivity (as opposed to gross functional abnormality) may be an associated finding in these patients, and acid suppression may lead to improvement in many patients.[22] The complex relationship between reflux and chest pain remains incompletely understood. Ambulatory pH monitoring, particularly during continued PPI therapy, remains the gold standard for diagnosis of GERD.

Associated GERD will be found in 70% to 80% of patients with asthma. Whether this finding represents cause and effect or the coincidental presence of 2 diseases is not clear. A careful history will reveal heartburn or regurgitation in only 50%. Onset of asthma late in life, the absence of a seasonal or allergic component, and onset after a big meal or alcohol consumption suggest GERD-related asthma. Empiric treatment with acid reflux suppression followed by pH testing in nonresponders has been suggested in one study as the most cost-effective means of determining whether GERD is aggravating a patient's asthma.[23] This approach seems reasonable, because it has been demonstrated that PPI therapy in asthmatic patients with gastroesophageal reflux improves peak expiratory flow rate and enhances quality of life.[24]

Reflux is the third most common cause of chronic cough, after postnasal drip and bronchitis, and the symptom of postnasal drip may actually be associated with reflux in many cases. Therefore, the prevalence of reflux as an etiologic factor in chronic cough may be even higher than has been recognized previously. GERD should be considered as the most likely diagnosis in the patient with cough, a normal appearance on chest radiograph, and no sinonasal postnasal drip.

Hoarseness is the most common otolaryngologic symptom of GERD. Most studies suggest that heartburn is present in only ≤50% of otolaryngologic patients with extraesophageal manifestations of GERD (such as hoarseness). However, some authors believe that a careful history may reveal heartburn to be present, at least occasionally, in as many as 75%.[25] Other associated symptoms of reflux laryngitis include halitosis, throat clearing, dry cough, coated tongue, globus sensation, tickle in the throat, chronic sore throat, and postnasal drip. Difficulty in warming up the voice in the professional singer, voice fatigue, and intermittent laryngitis are associated symptoms. Erosion of the dental enamel may be due to GERD; however, its frequency is not known.

COMPLICATIONS OF GERD

Patients with GERD may present with severe complications, including peptic stricture, ulceration, iron deficiency anemia, and, most important, Barrett's esophagus. Barrett's esophagus is a premalignant condition that involves a change from normal squamous epithelial lining to a metaplastic intestinal-type epithelium with typical special staining characteristics. Estimates are that 2% to 10% of patients with GERD will have esophageal strictures,[26] and 10% to 15% will have Barrett's esophagus.[4,27] Dysphagia, odynophagia (painful swallowing), and upper gastrointestinal bleeding may occur with these complications of GERD. Slowly progressive dysphagia, particularly for solids, suggests peptic strictures. Dysphagia for liquids and solids suggests a GERD-related motility disorder secondary to erosive esophagitis, Barrett's esophagus, or scleroderma. GERD-related motility disorders are seen with increased frequency in patients with otolaryngologic manifestations of GERD,[28] even though dysphagia is not usually a presenting symptom. Motility abnormalities pose important complications for the patient considering surgery (see Chapter 7). Odynophagia is uncommon in patients with reflux. Its presence suggests ulceration or inflammation, and it is seen most frequently in infectious or pill-induced esophagitis. Occasionally, esophagitis may present with occult, upper gastrointestinal bleeding or iron deficiency anemia. The frequency of these complications in patients with reflux laryngitis is not known.

GERD IS A CHRONIC DISEASE

There is ample evidence that patients with reflux esophagitis will experience endoscopic and symptomatic relapse up to 80% of the time if therapy is discontinued or drug dosage is decreased. Studies of patients with otolaryngologic manifestations of GERD suggest similar findings. Recurrence of hoarseness was seen within 6 months in one study.[29] The clinical impression is that GERD is chronic, with variable expression of this chronicity in different persons. Most patients, especially those with extraesophageal disease, require long-term medical therapy or surgery to achieve adequate symptom relief.

REFERENCES

1. Gallup Organization. *A Gallup Survey on Heartburn Across America.* Princeton, NJ: Author; 1988.
2. Dent J, El-Serag HB, Wallander, et al. Epidemiology of gastro-oesophageal reflux disease: a systematic review. *Gut.* 2005;54: 710–717.

3. Nebel OT, Fornes MF, Castell DO. Symptomatic gastroesophageal reflux: incidence and precipitating factors. *Am J Dig Dis.* 1976;21: 953–956.

4. Winters C Jr, Spurling TJ, Chobanian SJ, et al. Barrett's esophagus: a prevalent, occult complication of gastroesophageal reflux disease. *Gastroenterology.* 1987;92:118–124.

5. Ollyo JB, Monnier P, Fontollier C, et al. The natural history, prevalence and incidence of reflux esophagitis. *Gullet.* 1993;3(suppl): 3–10.

6. Pace F, Santalucia F, Bianchi Porro G. Natural history of gastro-oesophageal reflux disease without esophagitis. *Gut.* 1991;32:845–848.

7. Schnatz PF, Castell JA, Castell DO. Pulmonary symptoms associated with gastroesophageal reflux: use of ambulatory pH monitoring to diagnose and to direct therapy. *Am J Gastroenterol.* 1996;91: 1715–1718.

8. Harding SM, Richter JE, Guzzo MR, et al. Asthma and gastroesophageal reflux: acid suppression therapy improves asthma outcome. *Am J Med.* 1996;100:395–405.

9. El-Serag HB, Sonnenberg A. Comorbid occurrence of laryngeal or pulmonary disease with esophagitis in United States military veterans. *Gastroenterology.* 1997;113:755–760.

10. Koufman JA. The otolaryngologic manifestations of gastroesophageal reflux disease: a clinical investigation of 225 patients using ambulatory 24-hour pH monitoring and an experimental investigation of the role of acid and pepsin in the development of laryngeal injury. *Laryngoscope.* 1991;101(suppl 53):1–78.

11. Harding SM, Guzzo MR, Richter JE. Prevalence of GERD in asthmatics without reflux symptoms. *Gastroenterology.* 1997;4:A141.

12. Sontag SJ, O'Connell S, Khandelwal S, et al. Most asthmatics have gastroesophageal reflux with or without bronchodilator therapy. *Gastroenterology.* 1990;99:613–620.

13. Irwin RS, French CL, Curley FJ, et al. Chronic cough due to gastroesophageal reflux. Clinical, diagnostic, and pathogenic aspects. *Chest.* 1993;194:1511–1517.

14. Katz PO, Castell DO. Approach to the patient with unexplained chest pain. *Am J Gastroenterol.* 2000;95(suppl):S4–S8.

15. Hewson EG, Sinclair JW, Dalton CB, Richter JE. Twenty-four hour esophageal pH monitoring: the most useful test for evaluating non-cardiac chest pain. *Am J Med.* 1991;90:576–583.

16. Cherian P, Smith LF, Bardhan KD, Thorpe J, Oakley GD, Dawson D. Esophageal tests in the evaluation of non-cardiac chest pain. *Dis Esophagus.* 1995;8:129–133.

17. Larrain A, Carrasco E, Galleguillos F, et al. Medical and surgical treatment of nonallergic asthma associated with gastroesophageal reflux. *Chest.* 1991;99:1330–1335.

18. Sontag SJ, Schnell TG, Miller TQ, et al. Prevalence of oesophagitis in asthmatics. *Gut.* 1992;33:872–876.

19. Achem SR, Kolts BE, MacMath T, et al. Effects of omeprazole versus placebo in treatment of noncardiac chest pain and gastroesophageal reflux. *Dig Dis Sci.* 1997;42(10):2138–2145.

20. Fass R, Fennerty MB, Ofman JJ, et al. The clinical and economic value of a short course of omeprazole in patients with noncardiac chest pain. *Gastroenterology.* 1998; 115:42–49.

21. Achem SR, DeVault KR. Unexplained chest pain at the turn of the century. *Am J Gastroenterol.* 1999; 94:3–8.

22. Borjesson M, Albertsson P, Dellborg M, et al. Esophageal dysfunction in syndrome X. *Am J Cardiol.* 1998; 82:1187–1191.

23. O'Connor JF, Singer ME, Richter JE. The cost-effectiveness of strategies to assess gastroesophageal reflux as an exacerbating factor in asthma. *Am J Gastroenterol.* 1999;94:1472–1480.

24. Levin TR, Sperling RM, McQuaid KR. Omeprazole improves peak expiratory flow rate and quality of life in asthmatics with gastroesophageal reflux. *Am J Gastroenterol.* 1998;93:1060–1063.

25. Govil Y, Khoury R, Katz P, et al. Anti-reflux therapy improves symptoms in patients with reflux laryngitis. *Gastroenterology.* 1998;114:562. Abstract.

26. Spechler SJ. Complications of gastroesophageal reflux disease. In: Castell DO, ed. *The Esophagus.* Boston, MA: Little, Brown and Co; 1992:543–556.

27. Lieberman DA, Oehlke M, Helfand M. Risk factors for Barrett's esophagus in community-based practice. *Am J Gastroenterol.* 1997;92: 1293–1297.

28. Fouad YM, Katz PO, Hatlebakk JG, Castell DO. Ineffective esophageal motility (IEM): the most common motility disorder in patients with GERD-associated respiratory symptoms. *Am J Gastroenterol.* 1999;94:1464–1467.

29. Kamel PL, Hanon D, Kahrilas PJ. Omeprazole for the treatment of posterior laryngitis. *Am J Med.* 1994; 96:321–326.

6

Reflux Laryngitis and Other Otolaryngologic Manifestations of Laryngopharyngeal Reflux

Although a majority of otolaryngologists have recently acknowledged the importance of reflux in causing otolaryngologic disease, the association has been recognized for more than 2 decades.[1–33] Otolaryngologists are becoming increasingly diligent in looking for erythema and edema of the mucosa overlying the arytenoid cartilages, in suspecting laryngopharyngeal reflux (LPR) as the underlying problem, and in treating this problem as the primary approach to therapy for various reflux-related conditions. However, the most recent evidence indicates that the entity of LPR represents a complex spectrum of abnormalities, and it is important for physicians to understand the latest concepts in the relevant basic science and clinical care of patients with LPR. Symptoms and signs related to reflux have been identified in 4% to 10% of all patients seen by otolaryngologists,[19,34–36] and it is probable that these estimates are low. Among patients with laryngeal and voice disorders, LPR appears to be strongly associated with, or a significant etiologic cofactor in, about half of these patients. Many of the current concepts regarding reflux laryngitis and related controversies have been reviewed recently in the otolaryngologic and gastroenterologic literature.[37–39]

SYMPTOMS, SIGNS, AND PHYSICAL EXAMINATION

Common symptoms and signs of reflux laryngitis include morning hoarseness, prolonged voice warm-up time (>20–30 min), halitosis, excessive phlegm, frequent throat clearing, xerostomia (dry mouth), coated tongue, sensation of a lump in the throat (globus sensation), throat tickle, dysphagia, regurgitation of gastric contents, chronic sore throat, possibly geographic tongue, nocturnal cough, chronic or recurrent cough, difficulty breathing (especially at night), aspiration, occasionally pneumonia, closing of the airway (laryngospasm), poorly controlled asthma, recurrent airway problems in infants, and occasionally dyspepsia (epigastric discomfort) or pyrosis (heartburn). However, in both our experience and that of others,[12,16,19] dyspepsia and pyrosis are frequently absent because patients with LPR do not develop esophagitis. Ossakow et al[12] studied reflux symptoms in 36 gastrointestinal (GI) patients and 63 otorhinolaryngologic (ORL) patients. In their population, none of the GI patients had hoarseness, but all of the ORL patients complained of hoarseness. Only 6% of the ORL patients had heartburn; however, heartburn was reported in 89% of the GI patients. This low prevalence of heartburn is consistent with our experience. In a particularly important study, Wiener et al[16] evaluated 32 patients with hoarseness. Esophageal manometry findings were normal in all 32 patients.

Of importance, although pH monitoring study findings were abnormal in 78%, esophageal biopsy findings were normal in 72%. These results highlight the important fact that gastric acid can reflux through the esophagus to the larynx without causing esophageal injury in transit. Koufman's data on patients undergoing barium esophagram revealed that only 18% of patients with LPR had esophagitis identified on barium study,[19] although the barium swallow study is a very insensitive test for esophagitis. Presumably, the incidence of esophagitis is relatively low because distal esophageal mucosa has specialization and defense mechanisms that help it tolerate acid exposure.

Esophageal protective mechanisms include peristalsis, which clears acid from the esophagus; a mucosal structure that may be specialized to tolerate intermittent acid contact; the acid-neutralizing capacity of saliva that passes through the esophagus[40]; and bicarbonate production in the esophagus, which has been recognized since the 1980s.[41,42] Of interest, however, is that if some patients stop reflux treatment after a few months, classic dyspepsia and pyrosis seem to be present commonly when symptoms recur, although this clinically observed phenomenon has not been studied formally. It should be noted that the larynx and pharynx do not have protective mechanisms against mucosal injury such as those found in the esophagus. Thus, exposure to acid and pepsin that may be of no consequence in the distal esophagus may cause substantial symptoms and signs in the larynx and/or pharynx of some patients. Preliminary data reported by Axford et al[43] suggest that laryngeal mucosa has different cellular defenses from those of esophageal mucosa. These investigators also suggested that there may be specific differences in mucin gene expression and carbonic anhydrase, suggesting a pattern of abnormality in patients with LPR.

In addition to prolonged vocal warm-up time, professional singers and actors may also complain of vocal practice interference, manifested by frequent throat clearing and excessive phlegm, especially during the first 10 to 20 minutes of vocal exercises or singing. Hyperfunctional technique during speaking and especially singing is also associated with reflux laryngitis, which is probably due to the vocalist's unconscious tendency to guard against aspiration. Voice professionals can be helped somewhat in overcoming this secondary muscular tension dysphonia through voice therapy with speech-language pathologists, singing voice specialists, and acting voice specialists, but it is difficult to overcome completely until excellent reflux control has been achieved.

In addition to the paucity of typical gastroesophageal reflux disease (GERD) symptoms in patients with LPR, the tendency to underdiagnose LPR has been increased by 3 additional factors. First, the importance of various aspects of the physical examination is underappreciated. Posterior laryngitis and interarytenoid pachydermia are frequently ignored. It is even more common to fail to recognize the causal relationship between reflux and edema with little or no erythema, especially if the edema is diffuse, rather than most prominent on the arytenoids. Second, therapeutic medication trials may fail because patients are undermedicated (eg, with a proton-pump inhibitor [PPI] given only once daily) or assessed before signs of LPR have had time to resolve (which may require a few months or more). Third, results of routine tests for GERD can be falsely negative. This problem involves not only barium esophagrams, the Bernstein acid-hyperperfusion test, and radionuclide scanning but also esophagoscopy and 24-hour pH monitoring studies (depending on the norms used). Consequently, laryngologists must maintain a high index of suspicion in the presence of symptoms consistent with LPR, evaluate such patients aggressively, and interpret test results knowledgeably and with awareness of their sensitivities, specificities, limitations, and controversies.

Physical examination of patients with throat and voice complaints must be comprehensive. A thorough head and neck examination is always included, with particular attention paid to the ears and hearing, nasal patency, signs of allergy, the oral cavity, temporomandibular joints, the larynx, and the neck. In some patients with LPR severe enough to involve the oral cavity, there is also loss of dental enamel. Hence, transparency of the lower portion of the central incisors may be seen occasionally in reflux patients, although it may be more common in patients with bulimia and those who habitually eat lemons. At least a limited general physical examination is conducted to look for signs of systemic disease that may present as throat or voice complaints. More comprehensive specialized physical examinations by medical consultants should be sought when indicated.

When the patient complains of vocal difficulties, laryngeal examination is mandatory. It should be performed initially using a mirror or flexible fiber-optic laryngoscope, but comprehensive laryngeal examination requires strobovideolaryngoscopy for slow-motion evaluation of the vibratory margin of the vocal folds. Formal assessment of the speaking voice and singing voice also should be performed, when appropriate. Objective voice analysis quantifies voice quality, pulmonary function, valvular efficiency of the vocal folds, and harmonic spectral characteristics. The neuromuscular function can be measured by laryngeal electromyography. These aspects of the physical examination and tests of voice function are discussed elsewhere and are not reviewed in this chapter.

Most commonly, laryngoscopy in patients with LPR reveals erythema and edema. Classically, reflux laryngitis involves erythema of the arytenoid cartilages and frequently interarytenoid pachydermia (a knobby or cobblestone appearance), as well as other signs[44] (Figure 6–1). However, many additional features may be observed, including edema of the false and true vocal folds, partial effacement or obliteration of the laryngeal ventricle, pseudosulcus (a longitudinal groove extending below the vibratory margin throughout the length of the vocal fold, including the cartilaginous portion), Reinke's edema, granulomas or ulcers (most commonly in the region of the vocal process), nodules and other masses, an interarytenoid bar, laryngeal stenosis, and other abnormalities. Koufman et al[45] reported that edema was even slightly more common than erythema: edema was diagnosed in 89% of 46 patients, compared with 87% who had erythema, 19% with granuloma or granulation tissue, and 2% with ulceration.

Belafsky et al[46] developed a reflux finding score that rates signs and appears to correlate with the presence of LPR. They advocate use of this instrument in combination with the reflux symptom index.[47] The reflux finding score depends on observations of subglottic edema, ventricular obliteration, erythema/hyperemia, vocal fold edema, diffuse laryngeal edema, posterior laryngeal hypertrophy, granuloma/granulation tissue, and thick endolaryngeal mucus. Although additional research from other centers is needed to confirm the validity and reliability of the reflux finding score, the authors found excellent inter- and intraobserver reproducibility (although all observers were practicing at the same medical center); they found the reflux finding score to be an accurate instrument for documenting treatment efficacy in patients with LPR.

In patients with severe LPR, the finding of a hyperactive gag reflex is also common; of interest, they may also have decreased laryngeal sensation. One of us (R.T.S.) has performed functional endoscopic evaluation of sensory threshold testing on patients with LPR and found that responses were diminished prior to treatment and were improved following treatment. These findings are consistent with preliminary observations by Jonathan Aviv, MD (personal communication, 2000).

It should be noted that controversy exists regarding the significance of laryngeal findings. Credible studies of the sensitivity and specificity of laryngoscopy for diagnosis of LPR are needed, although a few initial reports exist in the literature. Carr et al[48] studied 155 children retrospectively. In a chart review of direct laryngoscopy and bronchoscopy findings, they reported a positive predictive value of 100% for the combination of posterior chronic edema with any vocal fold or ventricular abnormality.

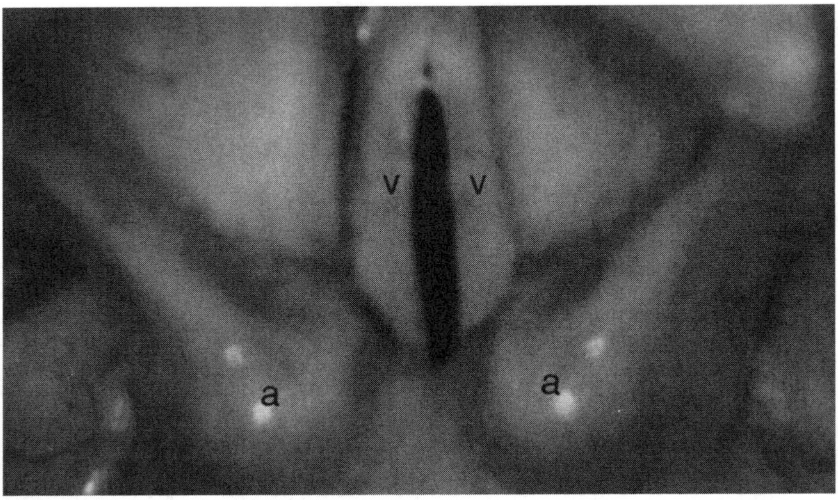

A

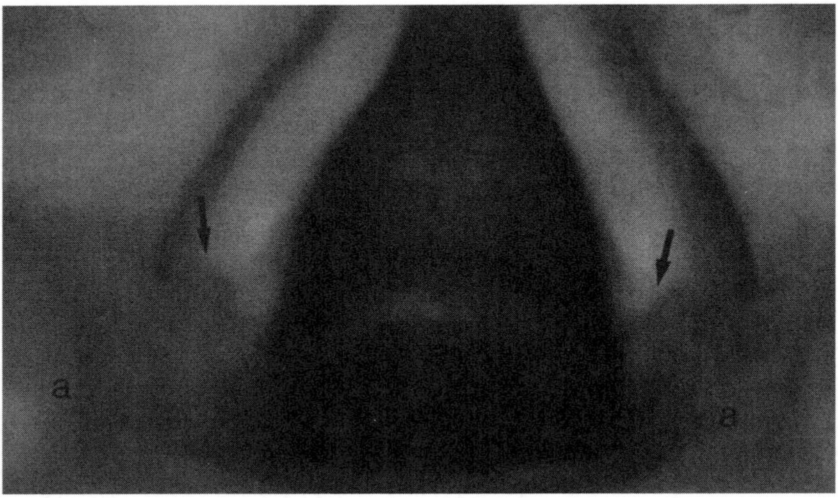

B

Figure 6–1. A. Normal laryngoscopic appearance showing the vocal folds (*v*) and arytenoids (*a*). **B.** Typical laryngoscopic findings in a patient with gastroesophageal reflux laryngitis. Note the marked arytenoid erythema (*a*), which extends as hyperemia of the posterior portions of the vocal folds (*arrows*). (A and B from Sataloff RT, *Professional Voice: The Science and Art of Clinical Care*. 3rd ed. San Diego, CA: Plural Publishing; 2005.) *(continues)*

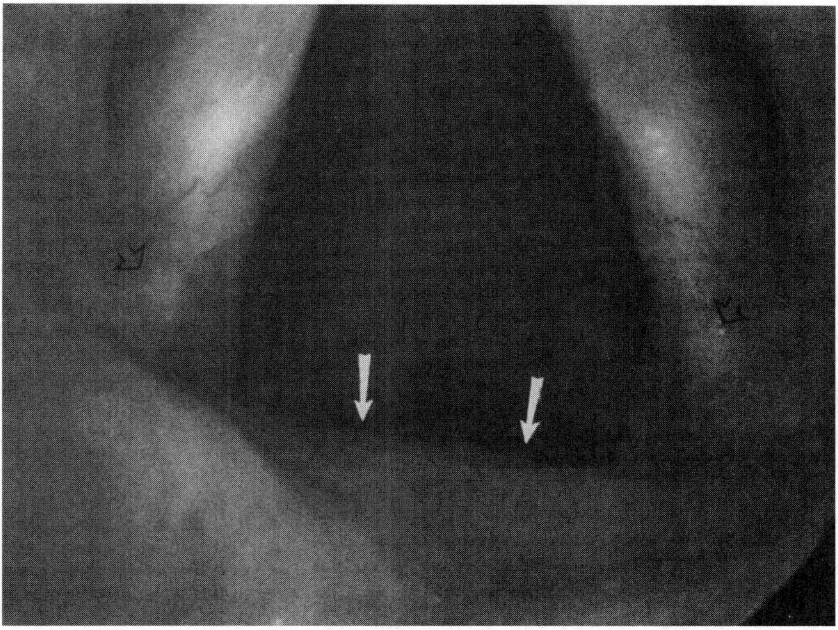

C

Figure 6–1. *(continued)* **C.** Laryngoscopic appearance in a patient with reflux and pachydermia (cobblestoning) involving the interarytenoid region (*white arrows*) and extending toward the cartilaginous portion of the larynx (*open arrows*).

McMurray et al[49] evaluated 39 children prospectively with laryngoscopy, bronchoscopy, esophagoscopy, and pH monitoring prior to airway reconstruction. Full-thickness laryngeal mucosal biopsy specimens were obtained from the posterior cricoid area and the interarytenoid area, and esophageal biopsy specimens were obtained. These investigators were unable to demonstrate a correlation among pH probe data, laryngoscopic findings, and histologic findings. Hicks et al[50] studied 105 healthy, asymptomatic volunteers. On laryngoscopy, more than 80% had at least one "abnormal" finding, including (in order of frequency from most frequent to least) interarytenoid bar, medial arytenoid erythema, posterior pharyngeal cobblestoning, medial arytenoid granularity, and true vocal fold erythema. This study did not perform 24-hour pH monitoring or any other tests to rule out the presence of "silent" reflux as a cause of the laryngoscopic abnormalities.

Despite many articles exploring signs and symptoms of reflux, including those cited above and other recent literature,[51–66] evidence confirming the diagnostic significance of various complaints and findings is scarce and contradictory. This is due to various problems, including the lack of a standard definition of "normal" in populations being studied. Continued interdisciplinary discourse and multicenter studies should be encouraged to answer important questions regarding the sensitivity and specificity of the many findings associated commonly with laryngopharyngeal reflux, as well as the impact of laryngopharyngeal reflux on quality of life and general health.[67]

PATHOPHYSIOLOGY

Laryngeal abnormalities may be caused by direct injury or by a secondary mechanism. Direct injury is due to contact of acid and pepsin with laryngeal mucosa, resulting in mucosal damage.[26–32,68,69] Alternatively, irritation of the distal esophagus by acid may cause a reflex mediated by the vagus nerve, resulting in chronic cough and throat clearing, which may produce traumatic injury to the laryngeal mucosa.[9,10,32,33,70]

Researchers are attempting to delineate pathophysiology. To show LPR as an extraesophageal manifestation of GERD, Groome et al[71] hypothesized that GERD patients would have some LPR symptoms if the pathophysiology were truly common. Through a questionnaire administered to 1383 GERD patients, they determined that the prevalence of LPR increases with the severity of GERD.[71] Although based on nonstandard questionnaires, the finding suggests a relationship. A similar study sought to exclude other causes of laryngitis and found LPR in 24% of patients with reflux esophagitis. The presence of LPR was best predicted by age, hoarseness, and hiatal hernia.[72] A third study, strengthened by confirmed diagnoses of GERD and LPR with esophagogastroduodenoscopy (EGD) and 24-hour pH monitoring, respectively, similarly showed that when both GERD and non-GERD patients were treated with PPIs, laryngitis symptoms and signs improved in the GERD group only.[73] These studies seem to point toward a common pathophysiology, suggesting that laryngeal symptoms are indeed caused by acid exposure.

Bile reflux also may cause laryngeal irritation.[74,75] In addition, recent findings raise many new questions about the pathophysiology of LPR. For example, Eckley et al[76,77] report that decreased salivary epidermal growth factor may be associated with LPR and warrants further study; and Altman's discovery of a proton pump in laryngeal serous cells and ducts of submucosal glands is particularly intriguing.[78] It has been established that pepsin in the larynx results in depletion of carbonic anhydrase isoenzyme III (CAI III) and squamous epithelial stress protein (Sep70), 2 laryngeal protective proteins.[79,80] Pepsin is taken up by laryngeal cells and can be reactivated by a drop in pH, as seen in LPR. Pepsin is found in the esophageal mucosa of patients with Barrett's esophagus and in the laryngeal mucosa of those with LPR.[81] Interestingly, pepsin irreversibly affects CAI III at pH below 4 only in laryngeal, not esophageal, epithelium.[82] These laryngeal receptors for pepsin may be another future target for intervention. They also might explain the presence of symptoms and signs of LPR with weakly acidic reflux, as pepsin may be active to some degree at any pH between 3 and 6.5,[83] although a longer exposure time may be necessary at pH 5 to produce damage.[84] Possible pepsin activity at pH much above 5 remains controversial. Mucin gene expression is also found to be downregulated in the presence of pepsin.[85]

Animal studies have shown that acid combined with pepsin (acid-activated enzyme) compromises the integrity of the vocal fold epithelium. In 2010, Habesoglu et al[86] reported that rats exposed to an acidic pH in the presence of pepsin developed edema of the lamina propria, submucous gland hyperplasia, and muscular atrophy. Erickson and Sivasankar[87] reported that the epithelial barrier resistance of the vocal fold is compromised when exposed to acid and pepsin. They described transepithelial resistance as a marker of epithelial barrier resistance that measures the ability to restrict movement of solute and solvents. The authors pointed out that <3 episodes of reflux per week could injure vocal fold mucosa, in contrast to 0 to 50 reflux events daily that are considered normal exposure in the distal esophagus.

In 2009, Johnston et al[88] reported that pepsin invades the laryngeal epithelial cells by receptor-mediated endocytosis and that pepsin activity is maximal at a pH of 2.0. Bulmer et al[89] in 2010 showed that the effects of acid and pepsin exposure on porcine laryngeal mucosa were similar to the effects observed in the human larynx in patients diagnosed with LPR. Samuels and Johnston[90] reported that the presence of pepsin in the airway indicates reflux. However, they reported that there are only 2 methods used to identify pepsin in the airways: immunologic and enzymatic, both of which have advantages and disadvantages. Richter[91] stated that gastric acid combined with pepsin and bile salts is known to be causally related to the development of chronic esophagitis and Barrett's esophagus. In contrast, they reported that weak or non-acid refluxate has not been shown to cause damage to the esophageal or extraesophageal structures, including the larynx and the lungs.

Histopathologic inflammation and its association with the pathogenesis of esophageal and extraesophageal disease has been the subject of ongoing research. Some studies that have focused on histology have produced interesting findings. One found significantly increased CD8+ lymphocytes in the epithelium of patients with LPR, with proportionally more in the luminal epithelial layer. Additionally, nonclassical major histocompatibility complex (MHC) molecule expression was found to be involved in the response to refluxate, suggesting that relying upon classical markers may lead to erroneous conclusions about the response of laryngeal epithelium to reflux.[92] Wada et al[93] evaluated histopathologic inflammation of the upper esophagus in comparison with the lower esophagus. When compared with their control group, they found inflammation of the upper esophagus to be significantly greater in patients with abnormal laryngopharyngeal symptoms and significantly greater lower esophageal inflammatory histopathology in patients with classic reflux symptoms (ie, GERD).

Park et al[94] used transmission electron microscopy to examine cellular damage of the esophageal epithelium by gastric refluxate. They measured the intracellular space and quantified its dilatation. They compared 2 groups: patients who had LPR without GERD and patients who had LPR with GERD. They reported that the intracellular space of the esophageal epithelium was significantly more dilated in the LPR-with-GERD group. Amin and colleagues[95] reported that dilatation of intercellular spaces of esophageal epithelium is considered a specific marker in GERD. They studied a group of patients with LPR and sore throat in whom they found dilatation of intercellular spaces in oropharyngeal biopsy specimens. They also found dilatation of intracellular spaces in the laryngeal mucosa in animal models exposed to pepsin.

There are important pathophysiologic differences between LPR patients and GERD patients. For example, combined upright and recumbent or nighttime reflux is typical for GI patients with GERD. Upright reflux and regurgitation also are the least common pattern in this population. However, patients with LPR are more likely to experience upright reflux commonly throughout the day,[12,16,19,36] often even in the absence of supine reflux. We have observed some patients with LPR who experience reflux exclusively (and constantly) when they sing. Motility abnormalities have been demonstrated with higher frequency in patients with LPR, resulting in delayed acid clearance in one study.[96] In contrast, Postma et al[97] demonstrated that patients with GERD have significantly longer esophageal acid clearance times than those measured in patients with LPR. However, it is not unusual for LPR patients to have abnormal upper esophageal sphincter (UES) function. In 1978,

Gerhardt et al[98] showed that experimental instillation of acid in the distal esophagus in patients with esophagitis and in normal controls produces increase in UES tone. This phenomenon does not occur normally in many patients with LPR,[37] although an increase in resting UES pressure has been demonstrated in patients with reflux laryngitis.[96] In 2010, based on their research, Szczesniak and colleagues[99] suggested upregulation of the esophago-UES relaxation response as a possible mechanism in the pathophysiology of reflux laryngitis. They found that the UES relaxation reflex induced by rapid air insufflation of the esophagus is upregulated in patients with posterior laryngitis compared with healthy controls. They also found that this group of patients had a higher pharyngo-UES contractile reflex threshold, which is considered a mechanism of airway protection.

Vardouniotis et al[100] reported that a hypotensive lower esophageal sphincter (LES) is a significant pathophysiologic component of LPR, noting that complex molecular mechanisms involved in the function of the LES and genetic factors are involved in tissue protection from reflux. They reported that compared with the esophageal kind, laryngeal and pharyngeal mucosa is more susceptible to tissue damage from refluxate because the larynx is not protected by peristalsis or buffered by salivary bicarbonate. They reported that transforming growth factor–beta 1, which inhibits inflammatory response, has shown gene overexpression in postcricoid fibroblasts and that fibroblast growth factor 2 has shown decreased expression. Cheng et al[101] suggested that the microphage activation caused by gastric acid exposure should be considered also in the pathogenesis of GERD and aspiration-induced lung disease.

Chong and Jalihal[102] reported a greater percentage of LPR symptoms in patients with heterotrophic gastric mucosal patch (HGMP) of the distal esophagus. HGMP is ectopic gastric mucosa typically observed distal to the UES and thought to be congenital. Due to the fact that HGMP can produce acid, the authors suggest that this may be the etiology of LPR in some patients. In fact, in their study, patients with HGMP experienced LPR symptoms to a greater degree (73.1%) compared with their non-HGMP patients (25.9%).

Salminen et al[103,104] and others have reported that the endoscopic prevalence of HGMP is low, ranging from 0.1% to 10% in reported patients 16 to 75 years old. Typical symptoms in patients with HGMP include dysphagia, globus, pharyngeus, cough, hoarseness, and shortness of breath. They reported that the HGMP is a source of acid production, and have been supported by pH monitor studies showing gastic acid in this area. Parietal cells with oxyntic mucosa are the most common histologic type reported.

Laryngopharyngeal reflux can affect anyone, but it appears to be particularly common and symptomatic in professional voice users, especially singers. This is true for several reasons. First, the technique of singing involves "support" by the forceful compression of the abdominal muscles designed to push the abdominal contents superiorly and pull the sternum down. This action compresses the air in the thorax, thereby generating a force for the stream of expired air, but it also compresses the stomach and works against the LES. Singing is an athletic endeavor, and the mechanism responsible for reflux in singers is similar to that associated with reflux following other athletic activities, lifting, and other conditions that alter abdominal pressure, such as pregnancy (which is also influenced by hormonal factors). It has been established clearly[105] that reflux is induced by exercise even in asymptomatic, young volunteers (mean age, 28 y). Clark et al[105] demonstrated that running induced reflux more often than did exercise with less bodily agitation, such as bicycling, but both forms of aerobic exercise caused reflux, as did weight lifting in some patients. Postprandial exercise-induced reflux has a similar pattern, but with a greater amount of refluxate. It may be that the effect of exercise on reflux is even more pronounced in patients with GERD or LPR than it is in research subjects with no history of reflux symptoms, although this question has not been studied.

Second, many singers do not eat before performing because a full stomach interferes with abdominal support and promotes reflux. Performances usually take place at night. Consequently, the singer returns home hungry and eats a large meal before going to bed.

Third, performance careers are particularly stressful. Psychological stress has been associated with esophageal motility disorders (which may be associated with reflux) and with other gastroenterologic conditions, such as irritable bowel syndrome.[106] Psychological stress alone acts to increase the amplitude of esophageal contractions.[107] Stress may also affect the production of gastric acid. If psychological stress increases LPR, it may create a vicious circle. Pharyngeal stimulation may cause transient LES relaxation directly, or it may lower the threshold for triggering gastric distention.[108]

Fourth, many singers pay little attention to good nutrition, frequently consuming caffeine, fatty foods (including fast foods), spicy foods, citrus products (especially lemons), and tomatoes (including pizza and spaghetti sauce). In addition, because of the great demands that singers place on their voices, even slight alterations caused by peptic mucositis of the larynx produce symptoms that may impair performance. Thus, singers are certainly more likely to seek medical care because of reflux symptoms than are individuals with fewer vocal demands. However, careful inquiry and physical examination reveal similar problems among all patients. Most of the voice problems associated with reflux laryngitis appear to be due to direct mucosal damage from proximal reflux. The effects of distal reflux alone on laryngeal function have not been studied.

Voice abnormalities and vocal fold pathology may be due to reflux of gastric acid onto the vocal folds. Severe coughing may cause vocal fold hemorrhage or mucosal tears, sometimes leading to permanent dysphonia by causing scarring that obliterates the layers of the lamina propria and adheres the epithelium to deeper layers. Aspiration caused by reflux also makes reactive airway disease difficult to control. Even mild pulmonary obstruction impairs voice support. Consequently, afflicted patients subconsciously strain to compensate with muscles in the neck and throat, which are designed for delicate control, not for power source functions.[5,7] This behavior is typically responsible for the development of vocal nodules and other lesions related to voice abuse. Although it appears likely that some extraesophageal symptoms of reflux are due to stimulation of the vagus nerve rather than (or in addition) to topical irritation, the role of vagal reflexes in reflux laryngitis remains to be clarified.

POSTERIOR LARYNGITIS AND RELATED CONDITIONS

In addition to erythema and edema, more serious vocal fold pathology may be caused by reflux laryngitis. In 1968, Cherry and Margulies[26] recognized that reflux laryngitis is a potential causative factor in contact ulcers and granulomas of the posterior portion of the vocal folds, conditions that are discussed in detail later. They also observed that treatment of peptic esophagitis resulted in resolution of vocal process granulomas. Delahunty and Cherry[27] followed up on this observation by applying gastric juice to the vocal processes of 2 dogs and applying saliva to the vocal processes of a third dog that was used as a control. The control dog's vocal folds remained normal; the other dogs developed granulomas at the sites of repeated acid application. This experiment by Delahunty and Cherry is particularly interesting. The posterior portion of the left vocal fold of 2 dogs was exposed to gastric acid for a total of only 20 minutes per day, 5 days out of every 7, for a total of 29 days of exposure in a 39-day period. A total of 20 minutes out of 24 hours may not seem like an extensive exposure period; however, erythema and edema were apparent in both dogs by the fourth day of the first week. At the beginning of the second week, the larynges appeared normal after the 2-day rest period. However, visible reaction was provoked within 2 days after application was resumed, and the vocal folds never regained normal appearance. Marked inflammation, thickening, and irregularities were apparent in both dogs by the fourth week, and epithelial slough at the site of acid contact occurred on day 29 in one dog and on day 32 in the other. Granulation tissue appeared shortly thereafter. A similar procedure on a control animal was performed applying saliva to the vocal fold instead of gastric juice, and the vocal fold remained normal. This research suggests that even relatively short periods of acid exposure may cause substantial abnormalities in laryngeal mucosa.

Since that study, numerous authors have recognized the importance of reflux laryngitis as a causative factor in laryngeal ulcers and granulomas, including intubation granuloma.[1,2,7,26,109–115] In addition to its etiologic involvement in intubation granuloma, reflux laryngitis has long been recognized as a contributing factor to posterior glottic stenosis, especially following intubation.[116] Olson[113] has suggested that it may also be a causative factor in cricoarytenoid joint arthritis through chronic inflammation and ulceration, beginning on the mucosa and involving the synovial cricoarytenoid joint. We have encountered this problem as well. In addition to posterior glottic and supraglottic stenosis, subglottic stenosis has been reported as a complication of reflux.[3,117]

Laryngeal Granulomas

Laryngeal granulomas are a particularly vexing problem for both patient and physician. Granulomas, like contact ulcers of the larynx, usually occur on the posterior aspect of the vocal folds, often on or above the cartilaginous portion. They may be unilateral, although it is also common to see a sizable granuloma on one side and a contact ulcer on the other. Patients with ulcers or granulomas may complain of pain (laryngeal or referred otalgia), a globus sensation, hoarseness, painful phonation, and occasionally hemoptysis. Surprisingly, even large granulomas are often asymptomatic. On microscopic examination, these benign lesions usually contain fibroblasts, collagenous fibers, proliferated capillaries, leukocysts, and sometimes ulceration. Although the term "granuloma" is universally accepted, these laryngeal lesions are actually not granulomas histopathologically but rather chronic inflammatory lesions. However, granulomas and ulcers may mimic more serious lesions, such as carcinoma, tuberculosis, and granular cell tumor. Consequently, the clinical diagnosis of laryngeal granuloma must always be made with caution and must be considered tentative until the patient has been evaluated over time and a good response to treatment has been observed.

Understanding the etiology of laryngeal ulcers and granulomas is essential to clinical evaluation and treatment. Traditionally, ulcers and granulomas in the region of the vocal processes have been associated with trauma, especially intubation injury. However, they are also seen in young, apparently healthy professional voice users with no history of intubation or obvious laryngeal injury. In fact, the vast majority of granulomas and ulcerations (probably even those from intubation) are caused or aggravated by LPR disease. In some patients, muscular tension dysphonia producing forceful vocal process contact may be contributory or causal.

Evaluation of patients with laryngeal ulcers or granulomas begins with a comprehensive history and physical examination. In addition to elucidating specific voice complaints and their importance to the individual patient's life and profession, the history is designed to reveal otolaryngologic and systemic abnormalities that may have caused dysphonia. Special attention is paid to symptoms of voice abuse and of LPR, as discussed previously. It must be remembered that reflux laryngitis is commonly not accompanied by pyrosis or dyspepsia in these patients. The history also seeks specifically symptoms consistent with asthma, including voice fatigue following extensive voice use. Exercise-induced asthma can be provoked by voice use, and even mild reactive airway disease undermines the power source of the voice, which may lead to compensatory muscular tension dysphonia and consequent laryngeal granuloma or ulcer. Inquiry also investigates systematically all body systems for evidence of other diseases that may manifest with laryngeal pathology. It is important to include a psychological assessment. Excessive stress may lead to increased acid production, abnormal esophageal function, and symptomatic reflux and to muscular tension dysphonia. In such cases, it is important to identify and address the underlying stressor, as well as treat the symptomatic expressions of the stress.

Mirror examination usually reveals the presence of a granuloma or ulcer, but more sophisticated evaluation is invaluable. In the presence of suspected laryngeal granuloma or ulcer, one of us (R.T.S.) routinely performs strobovideolaryngoscopy using both flexible and rigid endoscopes. Flexible endoscopic examination reveals patterns of phonation and is extremely helpful in identifying muscular tension dysphonia and determining phonatory behaviors associated with forceful adduction. Some granuloma patients have a vocal fold closure pattern characterized by an initial forceful vocal process contact. Such a pattern implies an adduction strategy involving lateral cricoarytenoid muscle dominance—an important consideration in the treatment of granulomas that are refractory to therapy (medical and/or surgical) or those that recur. Rigid laryngeal stroboscopic examination provides magnified, detailed information of the lesions under slow-motion light, allowing analysis of their composition (solid granulomas versus fluid-filled cysts) and their effects on phonation. This examination also permits assessment of other areas of the vocal folds to rule out a specific lesion (eg, vocal fold scar) that may be the real cause of the patient's voice complaint.

Evaluation also includes at least a formal assessment by a speech-language pathologist skilled in voice evaluation and care. At our center, we also include objective voice analysis and a vocal stress assessment with a singing voice specialist (even with patients who are nonsingers). In addition to a laryngologist, a speech-language pathologist, and a singing voice specialist, evaluation by other members of the voice team may be indicated, depending on the patient's problems. Additional team members include an acting voice specialist, a psychologist, a psychiatrist, an otolaryngologic nurse clinician, a pulmonologist, a neurologist, a gastroenterologist, and others available for consultation. The information provided by these evaluations helps establish the degree to which voice abuse or misuse is present, and it guides the design of an individualized therapy plan.

Reflux must be suspected in virtually all cases of granuloma. Evaluation for this problem may include 24-hour pH monitoring, a barium swallow study with water siphonage (routine barium swallow studies are not satisfactory for diagnosing reflux, and the accuracy of barium swallow even with water siphonage is debatable), other tests, and a therapeutic trial of medical management. If there is historical evidence of prolonged reflux symptoms, endoscopic evaluation to rule out Barrett's esophagus is often advisable. It may be appropriate to biopsy the presumed granuloma at the same time. If a therapeutic trial of medications without confirmatory tests is elected, marked relief of symptoms and signs should occur following daily use of a PPI (before breakfast and dinner) within 2 to 3 months. Treatment for LPR should be aggressive.

The efficacy of oral corticosteroids for treatment of laryngeal granulomas and ulcers has not been proved, but they are used commonly on the basis of anecdotal evidence, especially for small or medium-sized granulomas and ulcers that appear acutely inflamed. For these conditions, low doses of steroids for longer periods are usually given, such as triamcinolone 4 mg twice a day for 3 weeks. Steroid inhalers are not recommended. They may lead to laryngitis or laryngeal *Candida* infections, and prolonged use may cause vocal fold atrophy.

At the end of 2 months of therapy including antireflux measures, voice therapy, and possibly steroids, substantial improvement in the appearance of the larynx should be seen. Ulcers should be healed, and granulomas should be substantially smaller. Patients should be examined after 1 month to be certain that the lesions are not enlarging. If they appear worse, biopsy should be performed promptly. However, it should be noted that complete healing may take 8 months or more.[118,119] Repeated strobovideolaryngoscopic examinations allow comparison of lesion size over time. If improvements are noted, aggressive therapy and close follow-up can be continued until the mass lesion disappears or stabilizes. If the mass does not disappear, or if response to the first 2 months of aggressive therapy produces no substantial improvement, biopsy should be performed to rule out carcinoma and other diseases. If the surgeon is reasonably certain that the lesion is a granuloma, injection of an aqueous steroid preparation (such as dexamethasone) into the base of the lesion at the time of surgery may be helpful. As long as a good specimen is obtained, the laser may be used for resection of suspected granulomas because the lesions are usually not on the vibratory margin, and they often are friable. However, one of us (R.T.S.) usually uses traditional instruments to avoid the third-degree burn caused by the laser (even with a microspot laser) in the treatment of this chronic, irritative condition.

It is essential that causative factors, especially reflux and voice abuse, be treated preoperatively and controlled strictly following laryngeal surgery. The patient is kept on therapeutic doses of a PPI prior to surgery and for at least 6 weeks following surgery. Surgeons can be comfortable using higher doses of PPIs (equivalent of omeprazole 40 mg twice a day before breakfast and dinner) as frequently as 4 times a day under these circumstances and, if necessary, adding a histamine-2 (H_2) receptor blocker (ranitidine, 300 mg) at bedtime. Following surgery, absolute voice rest (necessitating use of a writing pad) is prescribed until the surgical area has remucosalized. This is usually for ~1 week and virtually never longer than 10 to 14 days and sometimes as short as 48 hours. There are no indications for more prolonged absolute voice rest, although relative voice rest (limited voice use) is recommended routinely. Voice therapy is reinstituted on the day when phonation is resumed, and frequent short therapy sessions and close monitoring are maintained throughout the healing period.

As previously stated, granulomas recur in some patients. In all such cases, aggressive reevaluation of reflux with 24-hour pH monitoring studies is warranted because granulomas are seen commonly in patients with reflux laryngitis. Often, endoscopy with biopsy of esophageal and postcricoid mucosa is appropriate. Twenty-four-hour pH monitoring studies should be conducted with the patient off all medications except for a PPI or H_2 blocker. We have seen the rare patient "resistant" to PPIs who will demonstrate a normal gastric pH profile despite a dose of up to 80 mg of omeprazole daily or the equivalent dose of another PPI. Rarely some patients may demonstrate seemingly good response to PPIs initially, followed by loss of that response. In such patients, H_2 blockers may be effective. When medical management of reflux is insufficient, laparoscopic fundoplication can be considered for patients with recurring granuloma. Voice use must also be optimized and monitored with the ongoing help of the speech-language pathologist and with the assistance of other members of the voice team when indicated. The laryngologist and voice therapists must ensure that good vocal technique is carried over outside the medical office into the patient's daily life.

Occasionally, patients may develop multiple recurrent granulomas even after excellent reflux control (including fundoplication), surgical removal including steroid injection into the base of the granulomas, and voice therapy. Medical causes other than reflux and muscle tension dysphonia must be ruled out, particularly granulomatous diseases, including sarcoidosis and tuberculosis and neoplasms such as granular cell tumor. Pathology slides obtained at previous surgical procedures should be reviewed. When it has been established that the recurrent lesions are typical laryngeal granulomas occurring in the absence of LPR, the cause is almost always phonatory trauma. When voice therapy has been insufficient to permit adequate healing, some of these uncommonly difficult patient problems can be solved by temporary paresis of selected vocal fold adductor muscles (particularly the lateral cricoarytenoid) using injection of botulinum toxin (Botox; Allergan, Irvine, CA). Although this treatment approach has been effective, it is not utilized ordinarily for initial therapy and is appropriate only for selected cases.

Delayed Wound Healing

In addition to its possible carcinogenic potential, the chronic irritation of reflux laryngitis may be responsible for failure of wound healing. Reflux appears to delay not only the resolution of vocal process ulcers and granulomas but also healing following vocal fold surgery. For this reason, otolaryngologists are becoming increasingly aggressive about diagnosing and treating reflux before subjecting patients to vocal fold surgery, even for conditions unrelated to the reflux.

Stenosis

As noted previously, laryngeal stenosis has been associated with reflux.[3,19,28,37] Koufman[19] reported LPR in 92% of his patients with laryngeal stenosis, all of whom were documented by 24-hour pH monitoring studies. This finding is consistent with an earlier report by Little et al[28] in which the authors were able to produce nonhealing ulcerations and subglottic stenosis experimentally by applying gastric acid and pepsin to injured subglottic mucosa in canines. Long-term control of LPR is essential to success in treating laryngeal stenosis.

Globus Pharyngeus

The sensation of a lump in the throat, or globus pharyngeus, is associated commonly with LPR. The literature on the association of globus with reflux does not provide definitive guidance.[16–19,25,53,60,121–128] However, reflux has been found in 23% to 90% of patients with globus.[1,19,60,120–122,124,126]

Smit et al[125] studied 27 patients with globus pharyngeus alone, 20 patients with hoarseness alone (of >3 months' duration), and 25 patients with both globus and hoarseness. Using dual-probe pH monitoring, pathologic reflux was diagnosed if patients had a pH below 4 for more than 0.1% of the total time of monitoring, more than 0.2% of the time in the upright position, and more than 0% of the time in the supine position in the proximal probe or if they had more than 3 reflux episodes with pH below 4. The proximal probe was placed visually at the UES, and the distal probe was 15 cm from the proximal probe. Only 30% of patients with globus but without hoarseness had pathologic reflux. Smit et al found that only 35% of patients with hoarseness alone had pathologic reflux. However, 72% of patients (18 of 25) with globus and hoarseness had pathologic reflux. Sixty-five percent of patients with pathologic GERD had abnormal findings on esophagoscopy, including Barrett's mucosa in 2 patients. The diagnosis of LPR should therefore be considered in patients with globus pharyngeus, and diagnostic evaluation and a therapeutic trial of a PPI are warranted.[103] Similar findings were reported by Wilson et al (23%),[121] Curran et al (38%),[122] and Hill et al (30.8%).[124]

LARYNGOSPASM

Laryngospasm is forceful, involuntary adduction of the vocal folds. It is associated with airway obstruction that is often severe enough to cause feelings of panic in the patient. Typically, laryngospasm occurs suddenly and without warning. It may be precipitated by laughing or exercise, or it may occur with no apparent precipitating event. Nighttime attacks that awaken the patient are common. Reflux is a well-recognized cause of laryngospasm. The mechanism may be related to chemoreceptors on the epiglottis that respond to a pH of 2.5 or below by eliciting laryngospasm.[128] Loughlin and Koufman[129] also demonstrated that this reflex is dependent on a functioning superior laryngeal nerve. In our experience, LPR is the cause of paroxysmal laryngospasm in nearly all patients with this condition, and most respond to aggressive antireflux therapy.

Muscle Tension Dysphonia

The relationship between LPR and muscle tension dysphonia remains uncertain, but there is reason to consider an association possible. Koufman and coworkers[36] found a 70% incidence of LPR in patients with structural vocal fold lesions associated commonly with muscle tension dysphonia, including nodules, Reinke's edema, hematoma, ulcers, and granuloma. Chronic reflux laryngitis causes irritation that leads not only to an inflammatory response but also to laryngeal hyperirritability. Laryngospasm is the extreme manifestation of this condition. However, hyperfunctional posturing of the laryngeal muscles in response to chronic irritation or as a defense against unpredictably timed episodes of laryngeal aspiration of acid may conceivably lead to hyperfunctional patterns of voice use. Alternatively, in some patients LPR and muscle tension dysphonia may occur coincidentally, but injury to the vocal fold mucosa by acid and pepsin may make the vocal folds more prone to injury and to the development of structural lesions associated with phonotrauma. Traditionally, otolaryngologists and speech-language pathologists have viewed muscle tension dysphonia as a primary condition in the majority of cases. Our clinical experience (that of R.T.S.) suggests otherwise: a high percentage of patients with muscle tension dysphonia probably have an underlying disorder, such as reflux laryngitis or superior laryngeal nerve paresis, that may have been responsible for the hyperfunctional voice disorder. In all patients with voice abnormalities, including muscle tension dysphonia, it is essential to seek out and treat the primary etiologic condition.

Paroxysmal Vocal Fold Movement Disorder and Cough

Paroxysmal vocal fold movement disorder is a laryngeal dystonia characterized by intermittent glottic obstruction by adduction of the vocal folds on inspiration. It is also called paradoxical vocal fold adduction, respiratory dystonia, and other names, including paradoxical vocal fold movement disorder (PVFMD). Yelken et al[130] point out that PVFMD "mimics asthma," and patients are often diagnosed incorrectly initially. In their patients, they reported no relationship between asthma attacks and severity and PVFMD. However, they found LPR and allergy to be prevalent in their patients with PVFMD.

Cough associated with PVFMD was studied by Murry and colleagues.[131] They suggested that chronic cough associated with PVFMD might be due to laryngeal sensory deficits secondary to chronic acid exposure in the laryngopharynx, which triggers the cough reflex. They suggested also that the cough reflex could be an adaptive mechanism to clear particulate matter from the laryngopharynx.

Reinke's Edema

Prolonged acid or pepsin irritation of the laryngeal mucosa can result in significant alterations in laryngeal tissues, including carcinoma, as discussed in the next section. Reinke's edema appears to be one such tissue alteration. Koufman and Blalock[128] have demonstrated that abnormal 24-hour pH monitoring results in a majority of their patients with Reinke's edema, and this finding is consistent with our experience. In our opinion, it is unclear in many cases whether reflux is the primary cause of Reinke's edema or is a cofactor with other laryngeal mucosal irritants, such as smoking, hyperfunctional voice use, and hypothyroidism. However, we evaluate all patients with Reinke's edema for reflux and treat LPR aggressively. Many patients seeking optimal restoration of voice quality require surgical treatment despite good reflux control, voice therapy, smoking cessation, and correction of any thyroid abnormalities. Good reflux control should be maintained over the long term, but it is especially critical in the immediate postoperative period, as discussed previously in the section on delayed wound healing.

Carcinoma

The association of gastroesophageal reflux disease with Barrett's esophagus and esophageal carcinoma has been well established. It is now thought possible that LPR is associated with laryngeal malignancy as well.[132–136] Delahunty[4] biopsied the posterior laryngeal mucosa in a patient with reflux laryngitis and reported epithelial hyperplasia with parakeratosis and papillary downgrowth. In the 1980s, Olson[11]and others reported on patients (including young, nonsmokers, nondrinkers) with posterior laryngeal carcinoma in whom he believed reflux to be a cofactor. This issue also was addressed by Morrison,[137] who reported 6 cases of vocal fold carcinoma in patients who had severe reflux but had never smoked. In 1997, Olson[138] reaffirmed that the relationship between reflux and cancer is not conclusive.

The mechanisms by which reflux may cause laryngeal cancer remain speculative. Both smoking and alcohol consumption promote reflux by lowering pressure in the LES, impairing esophageal motility and mucosal integrity, increasing gastric acid secretion, and delaying gastric emptying. Accordingly, a high incidence of reflux in laryngeal cancer patients who smoke and drink is not surprising. However, the association does not explain how LPR may act as a cofactor in these patients or as a primary factor in patients who do not smoke and drink. Richtsmeier et al[139,140] have suggested that a deficiency in T cell–mediated immunity is causally related to immunodeficiency in cancer patients. There is a subgroup of suppressor T cells with H_2 receptors. Cimetidine, an H_2-receptor antagonist, inhibits the expression of suppressor T cells and enhances immune responses. Richtsmeier and Eisele[139] found that skin test anergy in laryngeal cancer can be reversed by cimetidine. This finding led Richtsmeier et al[140] to recommend the use of an H_2 blocker not only to treat reflux in laryngeal cancer patients but also to address their underlying immune dysfunction, although this thinking is not widely accepted.

Although some questions remain regarding the relationship between LPR and laryngeal carcinoma, the studies just cited, as well as more recent evidence,[141] suggest that the 2 conditions are probably associated. At present, patients with laryngeal cancer, or those at risk to develop laryngeal cancer, should be screened for reflux, and antireflux therapy should be instituted when it is present. Cancer surveillance is reasonable even in patients without known risk factors other than chronic LPR. The long-term efficacy of such treatment in prevention of malignancy remains unknown, but we have seen resolution of laryngeal structural abnormalities, including suspicious leukoplakia, in patients with LPR alone, and even in patients who continue smoking and consuming alcohol. Koufman and Burke[142] have reported similar experiences.

In 1988, Ward and Hanson[143] recognized reflux as a potential cofactor for the development of laryngeal cancer, particularly in nonsmokers. In 1991, Koufman[19] documented LPR in 84% of 31 consecutive patients with laryngeal carcinoma, only 58% of whom were active smokers. Freije et al[144] reviewed retrospectively 23 patients with T_1 and T_2 carcinomas of the larynx; they concluded that GERD plays a role in the etiology of carcinoma of the larynx, particularly in patients who lack typical risk factors (14 of their patients had quit smoking >15 years before developing laryngeal carcinoma), and may act as a cocarcinogen in smokers and drinkers. In 1997, Koufman and Burke[142] thought that the causal relationship between LPR and laryngeal malignancy remained unproved, but they noted that most patients who develop laryngeal malignancy have LPR, in addition to being smokers. Until more definitive data are available, we believe that long-term antireflux therapy in these patients merits consideration.

Studies have also examined the potential carcinogenic role of LPR. Conflicting data exist, complicated recently by published studies that show no carcinogenic effects but that were limited by short periods of acid injury.[145,146] Although some studies have shown LPR as a risk factor in animal models, others have not, and the true relationship between LPR and laryngeal malignancy remains uncertain. However, there are enough data indicating a possible link to suggest that at present, known reflux patients should be screened for laryngeal cancer and be made aware of this risk.[147]

Given the risk of esophageal adenocarcinoma in reflux patients, the value of EGD screening has been assessed. It has been argued that LPR symptoms are better indicators of esophageal adenocarcinoma than are gastroesophageal symptoms.[148] Studies have shown esophagitis in 12%–18% of LPR patients, and Barrett's metaplasia in 3% to 7%.[149,150] Additionally, in patients on long-term PPI, *Helicobacter pylori* is known to accelerate the loss of specialized gastric glands, causing atrophic gastritis and gastric cancer.[151] Serologic testing may screen for this infection. Diagnosis of hiatal hernia would also potentially affect treatment and is facilitated by EGD. Some have suggested routine EGD for patients complaining of heartburn; others suggest it for all LPR patients.[149]

Until the true relationship is defined, screening with either transnasal esophagoscopy or EGD (which may be performed at the time of routine colonoscopy in appropriate patients) is advisable. Many gastroenterologists are now advising visualization of the larynx during EGD. This has led to the diagnosis of LPR in up to 4.6% of patients undergoing EGD for GERD.[152]

Sudden Infant Death Syndrome and Other Pediatric Considerations

Laryngopharyngeal reflux is important in the pediatric population, although it has been studied much less extensively than has reflux in adults. Unlike adults, infants and young children are unable to complain of symptoms associated with LPR. Nevertheless, LPR has been associated with various problems in infants and children, including halitosis, dysphonia, laryngospasm, laryngomalacia, asthma, pneumonia, sleep apnea, and sudden infant death syndrome (SIDS).[19,153–179] The diagnosis can be established by laryngoscopy and bronchoscopy and by 24-hour pH monitoring studies. Children can be given H_2 blockers and/or PPIs, and fundoplication is appropriate in selected cases, particularly in patients with life-threatening complications of reflux.

Evidence suggests that SIDS may be causally related to acid reflux into the larynx. Hence, SIDS must join laryngeal and esophageal cancer at the top of the list of serious otolaryngologic consequences of reflux laryngitis. Wetmore[155] investigated the effects of acid on the larynges of maturing rabbits by applying solutions of acid or saline at 15-day intervals up to 60 days of age. Because the larynx not only is a site of resistance in the airway but also contains the afferent limb for reflexes that regulate respiration, he discovered that acid exposure resulted in significant obstructive, central, and mixed apnea. Gasping respirations and frequent swallowing were observed as associated symptoms. Central apnea occurred in all age groups but had a peak incidence at 45 days. Acid-induced obstructive apnea in rabbits is similar to obstructive apnea previously recognized in human infants with gastroesophageal disease. However, the demonstration of acid-induced central apnea produced by acid stimulation of the larynx is more ominous. Central apnea has been demonstrated in other animal models as a result of different forms of laryngeal stimulation. Central apnea resulting in fatal asphyxia has also been described in several animal models. Wetmore's study[155] suggests that gastroesophageal reflux alone is capable of triggering fatal central apnea. This possibility is particularly compelling when one recognizes that the peak incidence of central apnea occurring at 45 days in the rabbit corresponds well with the peak incidence of SIDS in humans, which occurs between 2 and 4 months of age.

Otolaryngologists should be aware of the prevalence of LPR/GERD in children and infants. Studies have shown that reflux is associated commonly with regurgitation and vomiting, disturbed sleep patterns, colic, gastrointestinal pain, croup, and hoarseness in the pediatric population.[180–182]

Monitoring of pH is valuable in infants with laryngitis, including pharyngeal monitoring, which may diagnose undertreated LPR or LPR missed on esophageal monitoring.[183] LPR is a known common cause of hoarseness in children and should be in the differential diagnosis.[184] It may be misdiagnosed as recurrent croup when reflux triggers intermittent airway obstruction.[185] The diagnosis of LPR is still often missed in children with hoarseness or frequent respiratory disorders.

In a recent study, Barreto et al[186] examined the laryngeal and phonatory effects associated with untreated growth hormone deficiencies. Values for roughness, breathiness, and strain were higher, and LPR signs were also more common in this population. More research is needed, but otolaryngologists should be familiar with this association.

OTHER CLINICAL PRACTICE CONSIDERATIONS

In treating LPR patients, the clinician is faced with management decisions centered on the entire aerodigestive tract. For example, the presence of pepsin in nasal lavage fluid has been documented in patients undergoing endoscopic sinus surgery.[187] LPR has been confirmed in these patients, suggesting a relationship between chronic rhinosinusitis and LPR. Nasal pepsin may also prove a future avenue of LPR screening.[187] Evidence also links LPR and chronic otitis media,[188] and surgical outcomes in laryngeal trauma surgery have proven better in patients with preoperative and postoperative PPI treatment.[189] Therefore, many different patient groups may benefit from reflux evaluation and treatment.

Pepsin has been found in tracheoesophageal puncture sites, as reported by Bock et al.[190] They performed tissue biopsy and collected secretions in 17 patients, 12 of whom had a history of GERD/LPR, and pepsin was detected in the majority of their patients. LPR also may play a role in the pathogenesis of dental disease and sleep disorders. Several studies have shown a relationship between LPR and dental erosion.[191,192] In an animal (rat) model study, Higo et al[193] identified microscopic dental erosion and loss of surface enamel secondary to regurgitation of acid, liquid, and gas, as well as destruction of teeth and supporting structures when they were exposed to gastric and duodenal contents. Ranjitkar et al[194] reported that casein phosphopeptide–amorphous calcium phosphate can protect teeth from erosion and damage caused by acid and bile products.

Becker et al[195] studied the role of LPR in patients with complaints of intraoral burning sensations. They placed an oropharyngeal pH monitoring probe at the level of the uvula and found no causal relationship between the symptoms of LPR and intraoral burning. They suggested that PPI therapy is not indicated in this patient population.

Researchers and clinicians have examined a myriad of symptoms in patients with LPR and the relationships between LPR and voice disorders, benign and malignant lesions in the larynx, chronic cough, pulmonary disease, asthma and allergy, and obstructive sleep apnea in both adults and children. Chung et al[196] examined the relationship between LPR and benign vocal fold lesions. They reported LPR in 65% of their control group, 66% of the vocal nodules group, 75% of the vocal fold polyp group, and 95% of the patients with Reinke's edema. Saleh[197] suggested links among reflux, postnasal drip, and chronic cough. Randhawa et al[198] pointed out that it is sometimes difficult to determine the cause of dysphonia, noting that the laryngeal findings on nasopharyngolaryngoscopy may be similar in patients with LPR and in those with allergy. In their small sample population, they diagnosed allergy in 10 patients and LPR in only 3 patients, which they felt raised the question of LPR being overdiagnosed.

Recent studies suggest a relationship between LPR and obstructive sleep apnea. Eskiizmir and Kezirian[199] suggested that the increased respiratory efforts used by patients with obstructive sleep apnea generate increased intrathoracic pressure, which contributes to increased reflux. Suzuki et al[200] suggested that relaxation of the LES might be the mechanism of reflux in patients with mild to moderate obstructive sleep apnea. They also found reflux-induced spontaneous arousals. Karkos and colleagues[201] reported that during sleep, UES pressures decrease significantly. However, they noted a lack of controlled trials and/or meta-analyses that address the correlation between reflux, snoring, and/or apnea. In 2010, Wang et al[202] examined the concentration of pepsin detected in oropharyngeal secretions in patients with LPR and obstructive sleep apnea. In the LPR population, they found higher levels of pepsin in sputum that correlated with a higher reflux symptom index and higher reflux finding score. In obstructive sleep apnea patients, they reported no relationship between pepsin levels and reflux symptom index.

Eryuksel et al[203] examined the relationship between LPR and chronic obstructive pulmonary disease. Before and following 2 months of PPI treatment, patients underwent laryngeal examinations and pulmonary function tests and were asked to complete questionnaires for LPR and chronic obstructive pulmonary disease. The authors reported significant improvement in chronic obstructive pulmonary disease symptom index and LPR symptoms and findings on laryngeal examination. De la Hoz and colleagues[204] studied reflux and pulmonary disease in 9-11 World Trade Center first responders. Their findings suggest that patients with reflux demonstrated reduced forced vital capacity, suggestive of air trapping and lower airway disease.

CONCLUSION

Treatment considerations in reflux patients are discussed in greater detail in Chapters 8 and 9. However, it should be emphasized that patients with reflux laryngitis frequently require more intensive therapy than is adequate for patients with dyspepsia in the absence of laryngeal symptoms and signs. In addition to monitoring symptoms and signs of reflux laryngitis, response to treatment is best judged by combined intraesophageal and intragastric pH monitoring of patients while they are receiving treatment. Such studies are worthwhile even when patients are taking PPIs, because rare patients continue to reflux acid on even high doses of PPIs,[205,206] and resistance to other PPIs may occur as well. Our recent observations suggest that omeprazole resistance also can develop in patients who respond well initially to the medication. Moreover, it must be recognized that normal results on a 24-hour pH monitoring study do not indicate the absence of reflux. Rather, such findings demonstrate the absence of acid reflux. Regurgitation of pH-neutral liquid may still be present and may produce symptoms, especially in singers and actors. Study of this phenomenon and its optimal management is badly needed.

Currently, although there are no data to support the superiority of surgery over medical therapy for LPR patients, it appears that selected patients may derive greater benefit from surgery than from medical management, especially when the efficacy and decreased morbidity associated with laparoscopic fundoplication, and the potential costs and risks associated with the use of H_2 blockers or PPIs for periods of many years, are considered. If endoscopic suturing and Stretta techniques prove efficacious, one or both of these techniques may be useful, but at present they have not been studied in LPR or compared with surgery or medical therapy.

Research into appropriate treatment regimens is ongoing, and extensive additional investigation is needed into the long-term effects of reflux on the larynx and on all the other mucosal surfaces above the cricopharyngeus muscle.

REFERENCES

1. Johnson LE. New concepts and methods in the study and treatment of gastroesophageal reflux disease. *Med Clin North Am.* 1981;65:1195–1222.

2. Ward PH, Zwitman D, Hanson D, Berci G. Contact ulcers and granulomas of the larynx: new insights into their etiology as a basis for more rational treatment. *Otolaryngol Head Neck Surg.* 1980; 88:262–269.
3. Bain WM, Harrington JW, Thomas LE, Schaefer SD. Head and neck manifestations of gastroesophageal reflux. *Laryngoscope.* 1983; 93:175–179.
4. Delahunty JE. Acid laryngitis. *J Laryngol Otol.* 1972;86:335–342.
5. Sataloff RT. The human voice. *Sci Am.* 1993;267:108–115.
6. Sataloff RT. Professional singers: the science and art of clinical care. *Am J Otolaryngol.* 1981;2:251–266.
7. Spiegel JR, Sataloff RT, Cohn JR, Hawkshaw M, Epstein J. Respiratory function in singers: medical assessment, diagnoses and treatments. *J Voice.* 1988;2:40–50.
8. Chodosh P. Gastro-esophago-pharyngeal reflux. *Laryngoscope.* 1977;87:1418–1427.
9. Hallewell JD, Cole TB. Isolated head and neck symptoms due to hiatus hernia. *Arch Otolaryngol.* 1970;92:499–501.
10. Ward PH, Berci G. Observations on the pathogenesis of chronic non-specific pharyngitis and laryngitis. *Laryngoscope.* 1982;92: 1377–1382.
11. Olson NR. The problem of gastroesophageal reflux. *Otolaryngol Clin North Am.* 1986;19:119–133.
12. Ossakow SJ, Elta G, Colturi T, et al. Esophageal reflux and dysmotility as the basis for persistent cervical symptoms. *Ann Otol Rhinol Laryngol.* 1987;96:387–392.
13. Kuriloff DB, Chodosh P, Goldfarb R, Ongseng F. Detection of gastroesophageal reflux in the head and neck: the role of scintigraphy. *Ann Otol Rhinol Laryngol.* 1989;98:74–80.
14. Lumpkin SM, Bishop SG, Katz PO. Chronic dysphonia secondary to gastroesophageal reflux disease (GERD): diagnosis using simultaneous dual-probe prolonged pH monitoring. *J Voice.* 1989;3: 351–355.
15. McNally PR, Maydonovitch CL, Prosek RA, Collette RP, Wong RK. Evaluation of gastroesophageal reflux as a cause of idiopathic hoarseness. *Dig Dis Sci.* 1989;34:1900–1904.

16. Wiener GJ, Koufman JA, Wu WC, Cooper JB, Richter JE, Castell DO. Chronic hoarseness secondary to gastroesophageal reflux disease: documentation with 24-hr ambulatory pH monitoring. *Am J Gastroenterol.* 1989;84:1503–1507.

17. Katz PO. Ambulatory esophageal and hypopharyngeal pH monitoring in patients with hoarseness. *Am J Gastroenterol.* 1990;85: 38–40.

18. Freeland AP, Ardran GM, Emrys-Roberts E. Globus hystericus and reflux oesophagitis. *J Laryngol Otol.* 1974;88:1025–1031.

19. Koufman JA. The otolaryngologic manifestations of gastroesophageal reflux disease (GERD): a clinical investigation of 225 patients using ambulatory 24-hour pH monitoring and an experimental investigation of the role of acid and pepsin in the development of laryngeal injury. *Laryngoscope.* 1991;101(4 pt 2 suppl 53):1–78.

20. Pesce G, Caligaris F. [Posterior laryngitis in the pathology of the digestive tract.] *Arch Ital Laringol.* 1966;74:77–92.

21. Vaughan CW, Strong MS. Medical management of organic laryngeal disorders. *Otolaryngol Clin North Am.* 1984;17:705–712.

22. Barkin RL, Stein ZL. GE reflux and vocal pitch. *Hosp Pract (Off Ed).* 1989;24:20.

23. Kambic V, Radsel Z. Acid posterior laryngitis. Aetiology, histology, diagnosis and treatment. *J Laryngol Otol.* 1984;98:1237–1240.

24. Jacob P, Kahrilas PJ, Herzon G. Proximal esophageal pH-metry in patients with "reflux laryngitis." *Gastroenterology.* 1991;100:305–310.

25. Wilson JA, White A, von Haacke NP, et al. Gastroesophageal reflux and posterior laryngitis. *Ann Otol Rhinol Laryngol.* 1989;98:405–410.

26. Cherry J, Margulies SI. Contact ulcer of the larynx. *Laryngoscope.* 1968;78:1937–1940.

27. Delahunty JE, Cherry J. Experimentally produced vocal cord granulomas. *Laryngoscope.* 1968;78:1941–1947.

28. Little FB, Koufman JA, Kohut RI, Marshall RB. Effect of gastric acid on the pathogenesis of subglottic stenosis. *Ann Otol Rhinol Laryngol.* 1985;94:516–519.

29. Gaynor EB. Gastroesophageal reflux as an etiologic factor in laryngeal complications of intubation. *Laryngoscope.* 1988;98:972–979.

30. Lillemoe KD, Johnson LF, Harmon JW. Role of the components of the gastroduodenal contents in experimental acid esophagitis. *Surgery.* 1982;92:276–284.
31. Johnson LF, Harmon JW. Experimental esophagitis in a rabbit model. Clinical relevance. *J Clin Gastroenterol.* 1986;8(suppl 1):26–44.
32. Cherry J, Siegel CI, Margulies SI, Donner M. Pharyngeal localization of symptoms of gastroesophageal reflux. *Ann Otol Rhinol Laryngol.* 1970;79:912–914.
33. von Leden H, Moore P. Contact ulcer of the larynx. Experimental observations. *Arch Otolaryngol.* 1960;72:746–752.
34. Koufman JA, Wiener GJ, Wallace CW, et al. Reflux laryngitis and its sequelae: the diagnostic role of ambulatory 24-hour monitoring. *J Voice.* 1988;2:78–79.
35. Toohill RJ, Mushtag E, Lehman RH. Otolaryngologic manifestations of gastroesophageal reflux. In: Sacristan T, Alvarez-Vincent JJ, Bartual J, et al, eds. *Proceedings of XIV World Congress of Otolaryngology–Head and Neck Surgery.* Amsterdam, Netherlands: Kugler & Ghedini Publications; 1990:3005–3009.
36. Koufman JA, Amin MR, Panetti M. Prevalence of reflux in 113 consecutive patients with laryngeal and voice disorders. *Otolaryngol Head Neck Surg.* 2000;123:385–388.
37. Koufman JA, Amin M. Laryngopharyngeal reflux and voice disorders. In: Rubin JS, Sataloff RT, Korovin GS, eds. *Diagnosis and Treatment of Voice Disorders.* 2nd ed. Clifton Park, NY: Delmar Publishing; 2003:381–392.
38. Ormseth EJ, Wong RK. Reflux laryngitis: pathophysiology, diagnosis, and management. *Am J Gastroenterol.* 1999;94:2812–2817.
39. Richter JE, Hicks DM. Unresolved issues in gastroesophageal reflux-related ear, nose and throat problems. *Am J Gastroenterol.* 1997;92(12):2143–2144. Editorial.
40. Helm JF, Dodds WJ, Hogan WJ, et al. Acid neutralizing capacity of human saliva. *Gastroenterology.* 1982;83:69–74.
41. Tobey NA, Powell DW, Schreiner VJ, Orlando RC. Serosal bicarbonate protects against acid injury to rabbit esophagus. *Gastroenterology.* 1989;96:1466–1477.
42. Hamilton BH, Orlando RC. In vivo alkaline secretion by mammalian esophagus. *Gastroenterology.* 1989;97:640–648.

43. Axford SE, Sharp N, Ross PE, et al. Cell biology of laryngeal epithelial defenses in health and disease: preliminary studies. *Ann Otol Rhinol Laryngol.* 2001;110:1099–1108.

44. Al-Sabbagh G, Wo JM. Supraesophageal manifestations of gastroesophageal reflux disease. *Semin Gastrointest Dis.* 1999;10:113–119.

45. Koufman JA, Wiener GJ, Wu WC, Castell DO. Reflux laryngitis and its sequelae: the diagnostic role of ambulatory 24-hour pH monitoring. *J Voice.* 1988;2:78–89.

46. Belafsky PC, Postma GN, Koufman JA. The validity and reliability of the reflux finding score (RFS). *Laryngoscope.* 2001:111:1313–1317.

47. Belafsky PC, Postma GN, Koufman JA. The validity and reliability of the reflux symptom index (RSI). *J Voice.* 2002;16:274–277.

48. Carr MM, Nguyen A, Poje C, et al. Correlation of findings on direct laryngoscopy and bronchoscopy with presence of extraesophageal reflux disease. *Laryngoscope.* 2000;110:1560–1562.

49. McMurray JS, Gerber M, Stenn C, et al. Role of laryngoscopy, dual pH probe monitoring, and laryngeal mucosal biopsy in the diagnosis of pharyngoesophageal reflux. *Ann Otol Rhinol Laryngol.* 2001;110:299–304.

50. Hicks DM, Ours TM, Abelson T, et al. The prevalence of hypopharynx findings associated with gastroesophageal reflux in normal volunteers. *J Voice.* 2002;16:564–579.

51. Close LG. Laryngopharyngeal manifestations of reflux: diagnosis and therapy. *Eur J Gastroenterol Hepatol.* 2002;14(suppl 1):S23–S27.

52. Tauber S, Gross M, Issing WJ. Association of laryngopharyngeal symptoms with gastroesophageal reflux disease. *Laryngoscope.* 2002;112:879–886.

53. Vaezi MF. Ear, nose, and throat manifestations of gastroesophageal reflux disease. *Clin Perspect Gastroenterol.* 2002;5:324–328.

54. Book DT, Rhee JS, Toohill RJ, Smith TL. Perspectives in laryngopharyngeal reflux: an international survey. *Laryngoscope.* 2002;112 (8 pt 1):1399–1406.

55. Branski RC, Bhattacharyya N, Shapiro J. The reliability of the assessment of endoscopic laryngeal findings associated with laryngopharyngeal reflux disease. *Laryngoscope.* 2002;112:1019–1024.

56. Noordzij JP, Khidr A, Desper E, et al. Correlation of pH probe-measured laryngopharyngeal reflux with symptoms and signs of reflux laryngitis. *Laryngoscope*. 2002;112:2192–2195.

57. Marambaia O, Andrade NA, Varela DG, et al. Laryngopharyngeal reflux: prospective study that compares early laryngoscopic findings and 2-channel 24-hour pH monitoring. *Rev Brasil Otorrinolaringol*. 2002;68:527–531.

58. Siupsinskiene N, Adamonis K. Diagnostic test with omeprazole in patients with posterior laryngitis. *Medicina (Kaunas, Lithuania)*. 2003;39:47–55.

59. Vaezi MF. Sensitivity and specificity of reflux-attributed laryngeal lesions: experimental and clinical evidence. *Am J Med*. 2003;115 (suppl 3A):97S–104S.

60. Issing WJ. Gastroesophageal reflux—a common illness? [in German]. *Laryngorhinootologie*. 2003;82:118–122.

61. Maronian N, Haggitt R, Oelschlager BK, et al. Histologic features of reflux-attributed laryngeal lesions. *Am J Med*. 2003;115 (suppl 3A):105S–108S.

62. Burati DO, Duprat ADC, Eckley CA, et al. Gastroesophageal reflux disease: analysis of 157 patients. *Rev Brasil Otorrinolaringol*. 2003;69:458–462.

63. Wang JH, Lou JY, Dong L, et al. Epidemiology of gastroesophageal reflux disease: a general population–based study in Xi'an of Northwest China. *World J Gastroenterol*. 2004;10:1647–1651.

64. Ahmad I, Batch AJ. Acid reflux management: ENT perspective. *J Laryngol Otol*. 2004;118:25–30.

65. Grillo C, Maiolino L, Caminiti D, et al. Gastroesophageal reflux and otolaryngologic diseases. *Acta Medica Mediterrancea*. 2004;20: 155–158.

66. Hill RK, Simpson CB, Velazquez R, Larson N. Pachydermia is not diagnostic of active laryngopharyngeal reflux disease. *Laryngoscope*. 2004;114:1557–1561.

67. Lenderking WR, Hillson E, Crawley JA, et al. The clinical characteristics and impact of laryngopharyngeal reflux disease on health-related quality of life. *Value Health*. 2003;6:560–565.

68. Chen MY, Ott DJ, Casolo BJ, et al. Correlation of laryngeal and pharyngeal carcinomas and 24-hr pH monitoring of the esophagus and pharynx. *Otolaryngol Head Neck Surg.* 1998;119:460–462.

69. Ludemann JP, Manoukian J, Shaw K, et al. Effects of simulated gastroesophageal reflux on the untraumatized rabbit larynx. *J Otolaryngol.* 1998;27:127–131.

70. Kjellen G, Brudin L. Gastroesophageal reflux disease and laryngeal symptoms. Is there really a causal relationship? *ORL J Otorhinolaryngol Relat Spec.* 1994;56:287–290.

71. Groome M, Cotton JP, Borland M, et al. Prevalence of laryngopharyngeal reflux in a population with gastroesophageal reflux. *Laryngoscope.* 2007;117:1424–1428.

72. Lai YC, Wang PC, Lin JC. Laryngopharyngeal reflux in patients with reflux esophagitis. *World J Gastroenterol.* 2008;14:4523–4528.

73. Qua CS, Wong CH, Gopala K, Goh KL. Gastro-oesophageal reflux disease in chronic laryngitis: prevalence and response to acid-suppressive therapy. *Aliment Pharmacol Ther.* 2007;25:287–295.

74. Galli J, Calo L, Agostino S, et al. Bile reflux as possible risk factor in laryngopharyngeal inflammatory and neoplastic lesions. *Acta Otorhinolaryngol Ital.* 2003;23:377–382.

75. Adhami T, Goldblum JR, Richter JE, et al. The role of gastric and duodenal agents in laryngeal injury: an experimental canine model. *Am J Gastroenterol.* 2004;99:2098–2106.

76. Eckley CA, Michelsohn N, Rizzo LV, et al. Salivary epidermal growth factor concentration in adults with reflux laryngitis. *Otolaryngol Head Neck Surg.* 2004;131:401–406.

77. Eckley, CA, Costa HO. Salivary EGF concentration in adults with chronic laryngitis caused by laryngopharyngeal reflux. *Rev Brasil Otorrinolaringol.* 2003;69:590–597.

78. Altman KW, Haines GK III, Hammer ND, Radosevich JA. The H+/K+-ATPase (proton) pump is expressed in human laryngeal submucosal glands. *Laryngoscope.* 2003;113:1927–1930.

79. Johnston N, Dettmar PW, Lively MO, et al. Effect of pepsin on laryngeal stress protein (Sep70, Sep53, and Hsp70) response: role in laryngopharyngeal reflux disease. *Ann Otol Rhino Laryngol.* 2006;115:47–58.

80. Johnston N, Knight J, Dettmar PW, et al. Pepsin and carbonic anhydrase isoenzyme III as diagnostic markers for laryngopharyngeal reflux disease. *Laryngoscope*. 2004;114:2129–2134.

81. Johnston N, Wells CW, Blumin JH, et al. Receptor-mediated uptake of pepsin by laryngeal epithelial cells. *Ann Otol Rhinol Laryngol*. 2007;116:934–938.

82. Johnston N, Bulmer D, Gill GA, et al. Cell biology of laryngeal epithelial defenses in health and disease: further studies. *Ann Otol Rhinol Laryngol*. 2003;112:481–491.

83. Johnston N, Dettmar PW, Bishwokarma B, et al. Activity/stability of human pepsin: implications for reflux attributed to laryngeal disease. *Laryngoscope*. 2007;117:1036–1039.

84. Ylitalo R, Thibeault SL. Relationship between time of exposure of laryngopharyngeal reflux and gene expression in laryngeal fibroblasts. *Ann Otol Rhinol Laryngol*. 2006;115:775–783.

85. Samuels TL, Handler E, Syring ML, et al. Mucin gene expression in human laryngeal epithelia: effect of laryngopharyngeal reflux. *Ann Otol Rhinol Laryngol*. 2008;117:688–695.

86. Habesoglu TE, Habesoglu M, Sürmeli M, et al. Histological changes of rat soft palate with exposure to experimental laryngopharyngeal reflux. *Auris Nasus Larynx*. 2010;37:730–736.

87. Erickson E, Sivasankar M. Simulated reflux decreases vocal fold epithelial barrier resistance. *Laryngoscope*. 2010;120:1569–1575.

88. Johnston N, Wells CW, Samuels TL, Blumin JH. Pepsin in nonacidic refluxate can damage hypopharyngeal epithelial cells. *Ann Otol Rhinol Laryngol*. 2009;118:677–685.

89. Bulmer DM, Ali MS, Brownlee IA, Dettmar PW, Pearson JP. Laryngeal mucosa: its susceptibility to damage by acid and pepsin. *Laryngoscope*. 2010;120:777–782.

90. Samuels TL, Johnston N. Pepsin as a marker of extraesophageal reflux. *Ann Otol Rhinol Laryngol*. 2010;119:203–208.

91. Richter JE. Role of gastric refluxate in gastroesophageal reflux disease: acid, weak acid and bile. *Am J Med Sci*. 2009;338:89–95.

92. Rees LEN, Pazmany L, Gutowska-Owsiad D, et al. Laryngopharyngeal reflux. *Am J Respir Crit Care Med*. 2008;177:1187–1193.

93. Wada T, Sasaki M, Kataoka H, et al. Gastroesophageal and laryngopharyngeal reflux symptoms correlate with histopathologic inflammation of the upper and lower esophagus. *J Clin Gastroenterol.* 2009;43:249–252.

94. Park S, Chun HJ, Keum B, et al. An electron microscopic study —correlation of gastroesophageal reflux disease and laryngopharyngeal reflux. *Laryngoscope.* 2010;120:1303–1308.

95. Amin SM, Abdel Maged KH, Naser AY, Aly BH. Laryngopharyngeal reflux with sore throat: an ultrastructural study of oropharyngeal epithelium. *Ann Otol Rhinol Laryngol.* 2009;118:362–367.

96. Fouad YM, Khoury RM, Hatlebakk, et al. Ineffective esophageal motility (IEM) is more prevalent in reflux patients with respiratory symptoms. *Gastroenterology.* 1998;114. Abstract 6506.

97. Postma GN, Tomek MS, Belafsky PC, Koufman JA. Esophageal acid clearance in otolaryngology patients with laryngopharyngeal reflux. *Ann Otol Rhinol Laryngol.* 2001;110:1114–1116.

98. Gerhardt DC, Shuck TJ, Bordeaux RA, Winship DH. Human upper esophageal sphincter. Response to volume, osmotic and acid stimuli. *Gastroenterology.* 1978;75:268–274.

99. Szczesniak MM, Williams RB, Brake HM, Maclean JC, Cole IE, Cook IJ. Upregulation of the esophago-UES relaxation response: a possible pathophysiological mechanism in suspected reflux laryngitis. *Neurogastroenterol Motil.* 2010;22:381–386.

100. Vardouniotis AS, Karatzanis AD, Tzortzaki E, et al. Molecular pathways and genetic factors in the pathogenesis of laryngopharyngeal reflux. *Eur Arch Otorhinolaryngol.* 2009;266:795–801.

101. Cheng CM, Hsieh CC, Lin CS, et al. Macrophage activation by gastric fluid suggests MMP involvement in aspiration-induced lung disease. *Immunobiology.* 2010;215:173–181.

102. Chong VH, Jalihal A. Heterotopic gastric mucosal patch of the esophagus is associated with higher prevalence of laryngopharyngeal reflux symptoms. *Eur Arch Otorhinolaryngol.* 2010;267: 1793–1799.

103. Salminen P, Ovaska J. Heterotopic gastric mucosal patch in patients with reflux laryngitis: an entity of clinical interest? *Surg Laparosc Endosc Percutan Tech.* 2009;19:361–363.

104. Basseri B, Conklin JL, Mertens RB, Lo SK, Bellack GS, Shaye OA. Heterotopic gastric mucosa (inlet patch) in a patient with laryngopharyngeal reflux (LPR) and laryngeal carcinoma: a case report and review of literature. *Dis Esophagus*. 2009;22:E1–E5.

105. Clark CS, Kraus BB, Sinclair J, Castell DO. Gastroesophageal reflux induced by exercise in healthy volunteers. *JAMA*. 1989;261: 3599–3601.

106. Castell DO. *The Esophagus*. 3rd ed. Philadelphia, PA: Lippincott; 1999:222–223.

107. Castell DO. *The Esophagus*. 3rd ed. Philadelphia, PA: Lippincott; 1999:582–583.

108. Castell DO. *The Esophagus*. 3rd ed. Philadelphia, PA: Lippincott; 1999:401.

109. Gould WJ, Sataloff RT, Spiegel JR. *Voice Surgery*. St. Louis, MO: CV Mosby; 1993.

110. Cherry J, Siegel CI, Margulies SI, Donner M. Pharyngeal localization of symptoms of gastroesophageal reflux. *Ann Otol Rhinol Laryngol*. 1970;79:912–914.

111. Goldberg M, Noyek A, Pritzker KP. Laryngeal granuloma secondary to gastroesophageal reflux. *J Otolaryngol*. 1978;7:196–202.

112. Ohman L, Olafsson J, Tibbling L, Ericsson G. Esophageal dysfunction in patients with contact ulcer of the larynx. *Ann Otol Rhinol Laryngol*. 1983;92;228–230.

113. Olson NR. Effects of stomach acid on the larynx. *Proc Am Laryngol Assoc*. 1983;104:108–112.

114. Teisanu E, Heciota D, Dimitriu T, et al. Tulburari faringolaringiene la bolnavii cu reflux gastroesofagian. *Rev Chir Oncol ORL Oftalmol Stomatol Otorrinolaringol*. 1978;23:279–286.

115. Miko TL. Peptic (contact ulcer) granuloma of the larynx. *J Clin Pathol*. 1989;42:800–804.

116. Bogdasarian RS, Olson NR. Posterior glottic laryngeal stenosis. *Otolaryngol Head Neck Surg*. 1980;88:765–772.

117. Fligny I, Francois M, Algrain Y, et al. Subglottic stenosis and gastroesophageal reflux [in French]. *Ann Otolaryngol Chir Cervicofac*. 1989;106:193–196.

118. Havas TE, Priestley J, Lowinger DS. A management strategy for vocal process granulomas. *Laryngoscope.* 1999;109:301–306.

119. Koufman JA. Contact ulcer and granuloma of the larynx. In: Gates G, ed. *Current Therapy in Otolaryngology-Head and Neck Surgery.* 5th ed. St. Louis, MO: CV Mosby; 1993:456–459.

120. Delahunty JE, Ardran GM. Globus hystericus: a manifestation of reflux oesophagitis? *J Laryngol Otol.* 1970;84:1049–1054.

121. Wilson JA, Pryde A, Piris J, et al. Pharyngoesophageal dysmotility in globus sensation. *Arch Otolaryngol Head Neck Surg.* 1989;115: 1086–1090.

122. Curran AJ, Barry MK, Callanan V, Gormley PK. A prospective study of acid reflux and globus pharyngeus using a modified symptom index. *Clin Otolaryngol.* 1995;20:552–554.

123. Shaker R, Milbrath M, Ren J, et al. Esophagopharyngeal distribution of refluxed gastric acid in patients with reflux laryngitis. *Gastroenterology.* 1995;109:1575–1582.

124. Hill J, Stuart RC, Fung HK, et al. Gastroesophageal reflux, motility disorders and psychological profiles in the etiology of globus pharyngis. *Laryngoscope.* 1997;107:1373–1377.

125. Smit CF, van Leeuwen JA, Mathus-Vliegen LM, et al. Gastropharyngeal and gastroesophageal reflux in globus and hoarseness. *Arch Otolaryngol Head Neck Surg.* 2000;126:827–830.

126. Malcomson KG. Radiological findings in globus hystericus. *Br J Radiol.* 1966;39:583–586.

127. Toohill RJ, Kuhn JC. Role of refluxed acid in the pathogenesis of laryngeal disorders. *Am J Med.* 1997;103(suppl 5A):100S–106S.

128. Koufman JA, Blalock PD. Functional voice disorders. *Otolaryngol Clin North Am.* 1991;24:1059–1073.

129. Loughlin CJ, Koufman JA. Paroxysmal laryngospasm secondary to gastroesophageal reflux. *Laryngoscope.* 1996;106:1502–1505.

130. Yelken K, Yilmaz A, Guven M, Eyibilen A, Aladag I. Paradoxical vocal fold motion dysfunction in asthma patients. *Respiratory.* 2009;14:729–733.

131. Murry T, Branski RC, Yu K, Cukier-Blaj S, Duflo S, Aviv JE. Laryngeal sensory deficits in patients with chronic cough and paradoxical vocal fold movement disorder. *Laryngoscope.* 2010;120:1576–1581.

132. Spechler SJ, Goyal RK. Barrett's esophagus. *N Engl J Med.* 1986;315: 362–371.

133. MacDonald WC, MacDonald JB. Adenocarcinoma of the esophagus and/or gastric cardia. *Cancer.* 1987;60:1094–1098.

134. Garewal HS, Sampliner R. Barrett's esophagus: a model premalignant lesion for adenocarcinoma. *Prev Med.* 1989;18:749–756.

135. Reid BJ. Barrett's esophagus and esophageal adenocarcinoma. *Gastroenterol Clin North Am.* 1991;20:817–834.

136. Chow WH, Finkle WD, McLaughlin JK, et al. The relation of gastroesophageal reflux disease and its treatment to adenocarcinomas of the esophagus and gastric cardia. *JAMA.* 1995; 274:474–477.

137. Morrison MD. Is chronic gastroesophageal reflux a causative factor in glottic carcinoma? *Otolaryngol Head Neck Surg.* 1988;99:370–373.

138. Olson NR. Aerodigestive malignancy and gastroesophageal reflux disease. *Am J Med.* 1997;103(5A):97S–99S.

139. Richtsmeier WJ, Eisele D. In vivo anergy reversal with cimetidine in patients with cancer. *Arch Otolaryngol Head Neck Surg.* 1986;112: 1074–1077.

140. Richtsmeier WJ, Styczynski P, Johns ME. Selective, histamine mediated immunosuppression in laryngeal cancer. *Ann Otol Rhinol Laryngol.* 1987;96:569–572.

141. El-Serag HB, Hepworth EJ, Lee P, Sonnenberg A. Gastroesophageal reflux disease is a risk factor for laryngeal and pharyngeal cancer. *Am J Gastroenterol.* 2001;96:2013–2018.

142. Koufman JA, Burke AJ. The etiology and pathogenesis of laryngeal carcinoma. *Otolaryngol Clin North Am.* 1997;30:1–19.

143. Ward PH, Hanson DG. Reflux as an etiological factor of carcinoma of the laryngopharynx. *Laryngoscope.* 1988;98:1195–1199.

144. Freije JE, Beatty TW, Campbell BH, et al. Carcinoma of the larynx in patients with gastroesophageal reflux. *Am J Otolaryngol.* 1996; 17:386–390.

145. Ling ZQ, Mukaisho K, Hidaka M, et al. Duodenal contents reflux-induced laryngitis in rats: possible mechanism of enhancement of the causative factors in laryngeal carcinogenesis. *Ann Otol Rhinol Laryngol.* 2007;116:471–478.

146. Del Negro A, Araujo MR, Tincani AJ, et al. Experimental carcinogenesis on the oropharyngeal mucosa of rats with hydrochloric acid, sodium nitrate, and pepsin. *Acta Cir Bras.* 2008;23:337–342.

147. Qadeer MA, Colabianchi N, Strome M, et al. Gastroesophageal reflux and laryngeal cancer: causation or association? *Am J Otolaryngol.* 2006; 27:119–128.

148. Reavis KM, Morris CD, Gopal DV, et al. Laryngopharyngeal reflux symptoms better predict the presence of esophageal adenocarcinoma than typical gastroesophageal reflux symptoms. *Ann Surg.* 2004;239:849–858.

149. Reichel O, Issing WJ. Should patients with pH-documented laryngopharyngeal reflux routinely undergo oesophagogastroduodenoscopy? A retrospective analysis. *J Laryngol Otol.* 2007;121:1165–1169.

150. Perry KA, Enestyedt CK, Lorenzo CS, et al. The integrity of esophagogastric junction anatomy in patients with isolated laryngopharyngeal reflux symptoms. *J Gastrointest Surg.* 2008;12:1880–1887.

151. Kuipers EJ. *Helicobacter pylori* and the risk and management of associated diseases: gastritis, ulcer disease, atrophic gastritis and gastric cancer. *Aliment Pharmacol Ther.* 1997;11(S1):71–88.

152. Katsinelos P, Kountouras J, Chatzimavroudis G, et al. Should inspection of the laryngopharyngeal area be part of routine upper gastrointestinal endoscopy? A prospective study. *Dig Liver Dis.* 2009;41:283–288.

153. Halstead LA. Role of gastroesophageal reflux in pediatric upper airway disorders. *Otolaryngol Head Neck Surg.* 1999;120:208–214.

154. Little JP, Matthews BL, Glock MS, et al. Extraesophageal pediatric reflux: 24-hour double-probe pH monitoring of 222 children. *Ann Otol Rhinol Laryngol.* (suppl)1997;169:1–16.

155. Wetmore RF. Effects of acid on the larynx of the maturing rabbit and their possible significance to the sudden infant death syndrome. *Laryngoscope.* 1993;103:1242–1254.

156. Landler U, Hollwarth ME, Uray E, et al. Esophageal function of infants with sudden infant death-risk [in German]. *Klin Padiatr.* 1990;202:37–42.

157. Kurz R, Schenkeli R, Hollwarth M, et al. Sleep apnea in infants and the risk of SIDS [in German]. *Monatsschr Kinderheilkd.* 1986;134:17–20.

158. Benhamou PH, Dupont C. Relationship between gastroesophageal reflux and severe malaise in infants [in French]. *Presse Med.* 1992;21:1673–1676.

159. Spitzer AR, Boyle JT, Tuchman DN, Fox WW. Awake apnea associated with gastroesophageal reflux: a specific clinical syndrome. *J Pediatr.* 1984;104:200–205.

160. McCulloch K, Vidyasagar D. Infantile apnea. *Am Fam Physician.* 1986;34:105–114.

161. Belmont JR, Grundfast K. Congenital laryngeal stridor (laryngomalacia): etiologic factors and associated disorders. *Ann Otol Rhinol Laryngol.* 1984;93(5 pt 1):430–437.

162. Jeffery HE, Rahilly P, Read DJ. Multiple causes of asphyxia in infants at high risk for sudden infant death. *Arch Dis Child.* 1983;58:92–100.

163. Camfield P, Camfield C, Bagnell P, Reese F. Infant apnea syndrome. A prospective evaluation of etiologies. *Clin Pediatr (Phila).* 1982;21:684–687.

164. Mark JD, Brooks JG. Sleep-associated airway problems in children. *Pediatr Clin North Am.* 1984;31:907–918.

165. Rosen CL, Frost JD Jr, Harrison GM. Infant apnea: polygraphic studies and follow-up monitoring. *Pediatrics.* 1983;71:731–736.

166. Haney PJ. Infant apnea: findings on the barium esophagram. *Radiology.* 1983;148:425–427.

167. Kahn A, Rebuffat E, Sottiaux M, et al. Sleep apneas and acid esophageal reflux in control infants and in infants with an apparent life-threatening event. *Biol Neonate.* 1990;57:144–149.

168. Ramet J. Cardiac and respiratory reactivity to gastroesophageal reflux: experimental data in infants. *Biol Neonate.* 1994;6:240–246.

169. Kahn A, Rebuffat E, Sottiaux M, et al. Lack of temporal relation between acid reflux in the proximal oesophagus and cardiorespiratory events in sleeping infants. *Eur J Pediatr.* 1992;151:208–212.

170. Paton JY, Macfadyen U, Williams A, Simpson H. Gastrooesophageal reflux and apnoeic pauses during sleep in infancy—no direct relation. *Eur J Pediatr.* 1990;149:680–686.

171. Paton JY, Nanayakkara CS, Simpson H. Observations on gastrooesophageal reflux, central apnoea and heart rate in infants. *Eur J Pediatr.* 1990;149:608–612.

172. Buts JP, Barudi C, Moulin D, et al. Prevalence and treatment of silent gastro-oesophageal reflux in children with recurrent respiratory disorders. *Eur J Pediatr.* 1986;145:396–400.

173. Rahilly PM. The pneumographic and medical investigation of infants suffering apparent life-threatening episodes. *J Paediatr Child Health.* 1991;27:349–353.

174. Sacre L, Vandenplas Y. Gastroesophageal reflux associated with respiratory abnormalities during sleep. *J Pediatr Gastroenterol Nutr.* 1989;9:28–33.

175. Vandenplas Y, Deneyer M, Verlinden M, et al. Gastroesophageal reflux incidence and respiratory dysfunction during sleep in infants: treatment with cisapride. *J Pediatr Gastroenterol Nutr.* 1989; 8:31–36.

176. Halpern LM, Jolley SG, Tunell WP, et al. The mean duration of gastroesophageal reflux during sleep as an indicator of respiratory symptoms from gastroesophageal reflux in children. *J Pediatr Surg.* 1991;26:686–690.

177. Graff MA, Kashlan F, Carter M, et al. Nap studies underestimate the incidence of gastroesophageal reflux. *Pediatr Pulmonol.* 1994; 18:258–260.

178. Gomes H, Lallemand P. Infant apnea and gastroesophageal reflux. *Pediatr Radiol.*1992;22:8–11.

179. Kurz R, Hollwarth M, Fasching M, et al. Combined disturbance of respiratory regulation and esophageal function in early infancy. *Prog Pediatr Surg.* 1985;18:52–61.

180. Singareddy R, Moole S, Calhoun S, Vocalan P, Tsaoussoglou M. Medical complaints are more common in young school-aged children with parent reported insomnia symptoms. *J Clin Sleep Med.* 2009;5:549–553.

181. Indrio F, Riezzo G, Raimondi F, Cavallo L, Francavilla R. Regurgitation in healthy and non-healthy infants. *Ital J Pediatr.* 2009;35:39.

182. Van Houtte E, Van Lierde K, Claeys S. Pathophysiology and treatment of muscle tension dysphonia: a review of the current knowledge. *J Voice.* 2011;25:202–207.

183. Ulualp SO, Rodriguez S, Cunningham S, et al. Pharyngeal pH monitoring in infants with laryngitis. *Otolaryngol Head Neck Surg.* 2007;137:776–779.

184. Block BB, Brodsky L. Hoarseness in children: the role of laryngopharyngeal reflux. *Int J Ped Otorhinolaryngol.* 2007;71:1361–1369.

185. Hoa M, Kingsley EL, Coticchia JM. Correlating the clinical course of recurrent croup with endoscopic findings: a retrospective observational study. *Ann Otol Rhino Laryngol.* 2008;117:464–469.

186. Barreto VM, D'Avila JS, Sales NJ, et al. Laryngeal and vocal evaluation in untreated growth hormone deficient adults (IGHD). *Otolaryngol HNS.* 2009;140:37–42.

187. Ozmen S, Yucel OT, Sinici I, et al. Nasal pepsin assay and pH monitoring in chronic rhinosinusitis. *Laryngoscope.* 2008;118:890–894.

188. Bercin S, Kutluhan A, Yurttas V, et al. Evaluation of laryngopharyngeal reflux in patients with suspected laryngopharyngeal reflux, chronic otitis media and laryngeal disorders. *Eur Arch Otorhinolaryngo*l. 2008;265:1539–1543.

189. Kantas I, Balatsouras DG, Kamargianis N, et al. The influence of laryngopharyngeal reflux in the healing of laryngeal trauma. *Eur Arch Otorhinolaryngol.* 2009;266:253–259.

190. Bock JM, Brawley MK, Johnston N, et al. Analysis of pepsin in tracheoesophageal puncture sites. *Ann Otol Rhinol Laryngol.* 2010; 119:799–805.

191. Cengiz S, Cengiz MI, Sarac YS. Dental erosion caused by gastroesophageal reflux disease: a case report. *Cases J.* 2009;2:8018.

192. Roth DF, Ferguson BJ. Vocal allergy: recent advances in understanding the role of allergy in dysphonia. *Curr Opin Otolaryngol Head Neck Surg.* 2010;18:176–181.

193. Higo T, Mukaisho K, Ling ZQ, et al. An animal model of intrinsic dental erosion caused by gastro-oeosophageal reflux disease. *Oral Dis.* 2009;15:360–365.

194. Ranjitkar S, Kaidonis JA, Richards LC, Townsend GC. The effect of CPP-ACP on enamel wear under severe erosive conditions. *Arch Oral Biol.* 2009;54:527–532.

195. Becker S, Schmidt C, Berghaus A, Tschiesner U, Olzowy B, Reichel O. Does laryngopharyngeal reflux cause intraoral burning sensations? A preliminary study. *Eur Arch Otolaryngol.* 2011;268: 1375–1381.

196. Chung JH, Tae K, Lee YS, et al. The significance of laryngopharyngeal reflux in benign vocal mucosal lesions. *Otolaryngol HNS*. 2009;141:369–373.

197. Saleh H. Rhinosinusitis, laryngopharyngeal reflux and cough: an ENT viewpoint. *Pulm Pharmacol Ther*. 2009;22:127–129.

198. Randhawa PS, Mansuri S, Rubin JS. Is dysphonia due to allergic laryngitis being misdiagnosed as laryngopharyngeal reflux? *Logoped Phoniatr Vocol*. 2010;35:1–5.

199. Eskiizmir G, Kezirian E. Is there a vicious cycle between obstructive sleep apnea and laryngopharyngeal reflux disease? *Med Hypotheses*. 2009;73:706–708.

200. Suzuki M, Saigusa H, Kurogi R, et al. Arousal in obstructive sleep apnea patients with laryngopharyngeal and gastroesophageal reflux. *Sleep Med*. 2010;11:356–360.

201. Karkos PD, Leong SC, Benton J, Sastry A, Assimakopoulos DA, Issing WJ. Reflux and sleeping disorders: a systematic review. *J Laryngol Otol*. 2009;123:372–374.

202. Wang L, Liu X, Liu YL, et al. Correlation of pepsin-measured laryngopharyngeal reflux disease with symptoms and signs. *Otolaryngol HNS*. 2010;143:765–771.

203. Eryuksel E, Dogan M, Olgun S, Kocak I, Celikel T. Incidence and treatment results of laryngopharyngeal reflux in chronic obstructive pulmonary disease. *Eur Arch Otorhinolaryngol*. 2009;266:1267–1271.

204. de la Hoz RE, Christie J, Teamer JA, et al. Reflux symptoms and disorders and pulmonary disease in former World Trade Center rescue and recovery workers and volunteers. *J Occup Environ Med*. 2008;50:1351–1354.

205. Bough ID Jr, Sataloff RT, Castell DO, et al. Gastroesophageal reflux disease resistant to omeprazole therapy. *J Voice*. 1995;9:205–211.

206. Klinkenberg-Knol EC, Meuwissen GSM. Combined gastric and oesophageal 24-hour pH monitoring and oesophageal manometry in patients with reflux disease, resistant to treatment with omeprazole. *Aliment Pharmacol Ther*. 1990;4:485–495.

7

Diagnostic Tests for Gastroesophageal Reflux Disease

The diagnosis of gastroesophageal reflux disease (GERD) is based normally on a combination of the patient's history, appropriate diagnostic tests, and relief of symptoms with carefully selected antireflux therapy. The patient presenting to the otolaryngologist poses special problems because the typical symptoms of reflux (heartburn and regurgitation) often are absent. When used appropriately, diagnostic testing with barium radiographic studies, esophagoscopy, laryngoscopy, esophageal motility testing, and ambulatory pH monitoring allows the clinician to demonstrate that reflux occurs, identify the end-organ effects of reflux (including esophagitis or laryngitis), confirm that symptoms are due to reflux, and evaluate upper esophageal sphincter (UES) pressure, lower esophageal sphincter (LES) pressure, and esophageal clearance. The approach to diagnosis of laryngopharyngeal reflux (LPR) in a general or otolaryngologic practice includes careful physical examination and diagnostic testing. This chapter discusses the use of each of these modalities in the management of GERD in general, with specific reference to the otolaryngologic patient (Table 7–1).

THERAPEUTIC TRIAL

When a patient presents with typical heartburn and regurgitation, diagnostic studies may not be needed. Relief of symptoms after a therapeutic trial with histamine-2 (H_2) antagonists, prokinetic agents, or

Table 7–1. Diagnostic Tests for Gastroesophageal Reflux

Is reflux present?
Barium swallow study
pH monitoring
Is there mucosal injury?
Barium swallow (air contrast) study
Endoscopy
Mucosal biopsy
Are symptoms due to reflux?
Therapeutic trial
pH monitoring (with symptom index)
Can prognostic or preoperative information be obtained?
Esophageal manometry
pH monitoring

proton-pump inhibitors for 8 to 12 weeks can confirm that the symptoms are secondary to GERD. Because heartburn is generally infrequent in the otolaryngologic patient, the end point of the therapeutic trial is dependent on other presenting symptoms; and diagnostic tests are often necessary to confirm the diagnosis. Historical clues that otolaryngologic symptoms may be due to GERD, specifically LPR, include, among others, morning hoarseness, halitosis, excess phlegm, dry mouth, and throat clearing.

If a therapeutic trial is used in a patient with suspected GERD and otolaryngologic symptoms, higher doses of antireflux agents, usually with a proton-pump inhibitor, for more than a few months periods of time are needed. However, neither cost-effectiveness nor clinical efficacy of any medical regimen in patients with LPR has been tested. We currently use a proton-pump inhibitor twice a day initially for a minimum of 8 to 12 weeks as a therapeutic trial for laryngeal symptoms suspected to be due to reflux. (See the section "Approach to the patient with otolaryngologic abnormalities related to GERD" in this chapter.) It must be remembered that a negative therapeutic trial does not necessarily mean that a patient does not have reflux. In some patients, symptoms are resistant to proton-pump inhibitors, and their reflux may not be controlled even when taking high doses of such inhibitors.[1,2]

Kotby et al[3] point out that the nonspecific clinical manifestations of LPR may be caused by other conditions and that there are a lack of well-controlled studies to assess response to treatment. We concur with their observations. Ayazi et al[4] reported that a meta-analysis of studies on the effects of proton-pump inhibitor therapy on controlling the symptoms of LPR suggests that only 50% of this patient population reports improvement in symptoms. However, we caution that intrinsic weaknesses in the meta-analysis raise concerns about the validity of the data. The authors proposed a new paradigm for diagnosing LPR based on loss of alkalization in the cervical esophagus. In their patients with LPR, they observed a failure to maintain a neutral pH in the cervical esophagus based on increased exposure to pH <4, and decreased exposure to pH ≥ 7, compared with normal patients. The authors suggested that sensitivity for detecting abnormal reflux and its causal relationship to laryngopharyngeal symptoms is increased by considering both the percent time recorded of pH <4 and the percent time with pH ≥ 7. They believe that loss of (inability to maintain) an alkaline (pH ≥ 7) environment in the cervical esophagus is an indicator of decreased ability to protect tissues from damage, in contrast to increased measurement of pH <4, which has been accepted as causing pathologic changes associated with LPR symptomatology. Chong[5,6] has suggested that the cervical inlet patch of the esophagus can be an etiology of LPR, but often it is unrecognized during endoscopy and subsequently underdiagnosed. He reported that the incidence of cervical inlet patch ranges from 0.29% to 10% in endoscopic examinations.

BARIUM RADIOGRAPHS

Barium studies are relatively inexpensive and widely available for use in the diagnosis of esophageal disease. When evaluating the esophagus, a double-contrast barium swallow is needed for optimal assessment. An upper gastrointestinal series usually results in insufficient evaluation of esophageal function, concentrates excessively on the stomach and duodenum, and does not give enough attention to potential mucosal or motility abnormalities in the esophagus. A hiatal hernia is the most common abnormality seen on barium swallow. However, hiatal hernia is present in up to 60% of the adult population,[7] making this a nonspecific finding and not diagnostic of GERD. Free reflux is seen in up to 30% of "normal" patients and may be absent in up to 60% of patients with GERD established by pH monitoring,[8] making the barium study insensitive and nonspecific for GERD. It has been suggested that reflux of barium to or above the carina or to the thoracic inlet is indicative of the potential for aspiration and is useful as an aid in the diagnosis of GERD-associated laryngitis. There are no prospective or controlled studies to substantiate this clinical impression. This finding is reported usually in studies performed with the patient in the supine position, making this observation of relatively little use. The so-called high reflux on a barium study has not been well correlated with proximal acid exposure on ambulatory pH monitoring. Barium swallow with water siphonage has been used to aid in the diagnosis of reflux in otolaryngologic patients. Patients may show abnormalities on barium swallow with water siphonage, which may be interpreted as confirming a diagnosis of pathologic reflux, although interpretations should be made with caution because the true positive predictive value has not been confirmed. However, barium swallow with water siphonage has more value than is recognized by many radiologists. The literature on this subject was reviewed in 1994 by Ott.[9] Because early reports revealed a wide discrepancy in reflux detection rates, barium esophagrams were considered insensitive, and provocative tests (such as water siphonage) were believed to increase sensitivity at the expense of specificity. Thompson et al[10] found that reflux detection rate increased to 70% when using the water siphonage test, compared with 26% for spontaneous reflux. However, this gain in sensitivity may be counterbalanced by the low specificity of the test.

In professional singers and actors especially, barium swallow with water siphonage seems to provide a good clinical approximation of daily reflux episodes. To optimize mucosal function, it is essential for singers and actors to remain well hydrated. Consequently they drink large amounts of water, routinely carry water bottles with them, and drink substantial quantities shortly before they sing. This routine behavior is similar to the water siphon portion of the barium swallow, which raises the question of whether a positive result on water siphonage tests constitutes useful information, at least in professional voice users, even when findings on 24-hour pH monitoring are normal. Specific mucosal abnormalities on double-contrast barium studies, such as thickening of esophageal mucosal folds, erosions, or esophageal ulcers, are seen in a minority of patients with GERD, making this study relatively insensitive for this diagnosis. The diagnosis of Barrett's esophagus is conclusive also by barium swallow.

The optimal use of the barium study is to evaluate patients with suspected complications of GERD such as motility abnormalities or peptic stricture, commonly seen in patients with solid or liquid dysphagia. A barium swallow can identify rings, webs, or other obstructive lesions, including carcinoma, seen in patients with dysphagia, but these are unusual complications of GERD. A solid bolus such as a marshmallow or a barium cookie can be given to help localize the site of obstruction in a patient with solid dysphagia.

Although the barium swallow allows demonstration that reflux is occurring and can demonstrate mucosal injury, it is of inconsistent value in establishing a diagnosis of GERD. Its best use is in evaluation of the patient with dysphagia, and it should be performed in conjunction with endoscopy in these patients. Nevertheless, in some patients, a barium esophagram provides important additional information that may be missed on radiologic imaging or esophagoscopy.[10–12] In a series of 128 patients, for example, barium studies showed esophagitis in 18%, a lower esophageal ring in 14%, and peptic stricture in 3%.[12] Consequently, patients with LPR should be considered for further evaluation by barium swallow if endoscopy is not planned.

RADIONUCLIDE STUDIES

Scintigraphic studies have been suggested as valuable in diagnosis of GERD.[13] A radioisotope (technetium-99m sulfur colloid) marker is mixed with a measured quantity of liquid (usually water), and graded abdominal compression is used to unmask reflux. Although radionuclide scanning was originally proposed as a sensitive test, its reliability has been questioned, and it is no longer considered a useful investigation.[14]

ENDOSCOPY

Endoscopy is used to document mucosal disease and establish a diagnosis of erosive esophagitis or Barrett's metaplasia. When patients with frequent heartburn and regurgitation are studied prospectively, erosive esophagitis is seen in 45% to 60%.[15] The remaining patients will have nonerosive disease (mucosal edema, hyperemia, or a normal-appearing esophagus). Erosive esophagitis suggests a serious form of GERD in which patients require continuous medical therapy with a proton-pump inhibitor or antireflux surgery for effective symptom relief and healing. Barrett's esophagus is seen in 10% to 15% of reflux patients undergoing endoscopy.[16] Unfortunately, there is no classic presentation of Barrett's esophagus, but it is most common in white males over 50 years of age.[17]

Erosive esophagitis is uncommon in patients with extraesophageal symptoms. Although 50% of patients with unexplained chest pain and normal coronary arteries have GERD, the prevalence of erosive esophagitis is 10% or less.[18] GERD-associated asthma and evidence of esophagitis on endoscopy have been reported in 30% to 40% of adult patients.[19,20] In patients with reflux laryngitis, erosive esophagitis is seen in only 20% to 30%, making this study of low diagnostic yield in GERD.[21]

Katsinelos et al[22] reported that the laryngopharynx is not examined routinely during esophagogastroduodenoscopy. Their prospective study found significant laryngeal pathology, including leukoplakia, Reinke's edema, and posterior laryngitis in their patients, and they recommended screening examinations of the laryngopharynx during all esophagogastroduodenoscopy procedures.

There are no absolute indications for endoscopy in the patient with suspected GERD. In general, endoscopy is performed in patients who do not respond to a therapeutic trial of medical therapy, patients with symptoms for longer than 5 years (to rule out Barrett's metaplasia), and patients with an "alarm" symptom of dysphagia: odynophagia, weight loss, anemia, or gastrointestinal bleeding.[23]

Although less useful today due to the widespread use of empiric proton-pump inhibitor therapy, endoscopic findings may help predict the prognosis and outcome of medical therapy. Patients with erosive esophagitis will almost always require long-term proton-pump inhibitor therapy for healing and symptom relief. Recurrence of erosive esophagitis is seen in up to 80% of patients within 3 to 6 months following the discontinuation of medications[24]; these patients usually require continuous pharmacologic therapy for effective long-term control. Because patients with nonerosive esophagitis seldom progress to more severe forms of esophagitis, patients with nonerosive disease can be managed with a range of pharmacologic treatments.

Since the introduction of the flexible endoscope, research and development have focused on improving image quality through changes in illumination, resolution, and magnification of images. Eller et al[25] compared fiberoptic and distal chip technologies using flexible laryngoscopy for recognizing laryngeal findings associated with LPR. Three senior otolaryngologists and 2 resident/fellow otolaryngologists were asked to grade physical findings of LPR on the images they evaluated using both a reflux finding score (see "Outcome measures" section) and a posterior erythema grading tool developed by the authors for this project. They compared the findings from these endoscopy systems with those from the images obtained with a rigid laryngeal telescope. The authors found that the fiberoptic and distal chip technologies were almost identical in their ability to detect LPR. However, both flexible technologies were found to be significantly less sensitive than a rigid laryngeal telescopic examination for diagnosing LPR.

New technology has been applied to video endoscopic systems, including narrowband imaging, iScan technology, and autofluorescent imaging.[26–35] High-speed optical coherence tomography can image cross-sections of soft tissue, and spectrally encoded confocal endomicroscopy provides images with subcellular resolution.[36–39] These technologies have shown great promise for advancing mucosal imaging and potential early detection of pathology.

Given the rarity of erosive esophagitis, we do not use endoscopy routinely as the initial study in patients with suspected GERD-related otolaryngologic disease, chest pain, asthma, or cough. We prefer ambulatory dual-probe pH monitoring or a therapeutic trial of antireflux medications as the initial diagnostic approach.

ESOPHAGEAL BIOPSY

Biopsy and cytology are of limited value in evaluation of the patient with GERD unless Barrett's esophagus or malignancy is suspected. The light-microscopic signs of GERD—elongation of rete pegs and hyperplasia of the basal cell layer[40]—do not distinguish between acute and chronic disease and do not help predict response to therapy. The microscopic signs of active esophagitis—polymorphonuclear leukocytes and eosinophils—are seen in a minority of adult patients,[40] so they are insensitive diagnostic findings. Biopsy may be more useful in the pediatric population, where a higher frequency of these findings has been reported.[41]

If Barrett's metaplasia is suspected, a systematic biopsy protocol should be followed to confirm the diagnosis and rule out dysplasia or carcinoma. Endoscopic surveillance with biopsies to rule out dysplasia is the current standard of practice for management of patients with Barrett's metaplasia.[42]

PROLONGED AMBULATORY PH MONITORING

Prolonged pH monitoring is the most important study to quantify esophageal reflux and determine whether symptoms are related to GERD. The study is most often performed in our laboratory using the transnasal approach. An antimony catheter (2-mm diameter) is positioned transnasally into the distal esophagus with an electrode placed 5 cm above the LES, which is identified by esophageal manometry. Precise positioning is important for accuracy in the interpretation of results. The probe is connected to a small microcomputer that is worn on a belt or clipped to the waist so that the patient can be monitored in an ambulatory setting. Activity can be tailored to provoke reflux in the setting in which symptoms are typically produced. For example, a patient with chronic hoarseness who sings professionally will be reminded to sing during the study. Some of our patients reflux constantly during singing, and rarely at other times (Figure 7–1).

Multiple electrodes can be placed on a single catheter to monitor intragastric and intraesophageal pH, distal esophageal and proximal esophageal acid exposure, or all of these simultaneously. Abnormal acid exposure in the proximal esophagus, just below the UES, predicts the potential for aspiration in patients with otolaryngologic symptoms. An intragastric electrode allows monitoring of the gastric acid response to antireflux therapy. Several investigators have placed probes above the UES in the hypopharynx[43,44] to document reflux above the UES in an attempt to confirm aspiration as the cause of symptoms. Muderris et al[45] suggested that a triple sensor pH catheter could accurately identify episodes of hypopharyngeal reflux when the proximal probe is placed in the pharynx and not in the upper esophagus. However, the accuracy of standard esophageal probes when placed in the pharynx has been

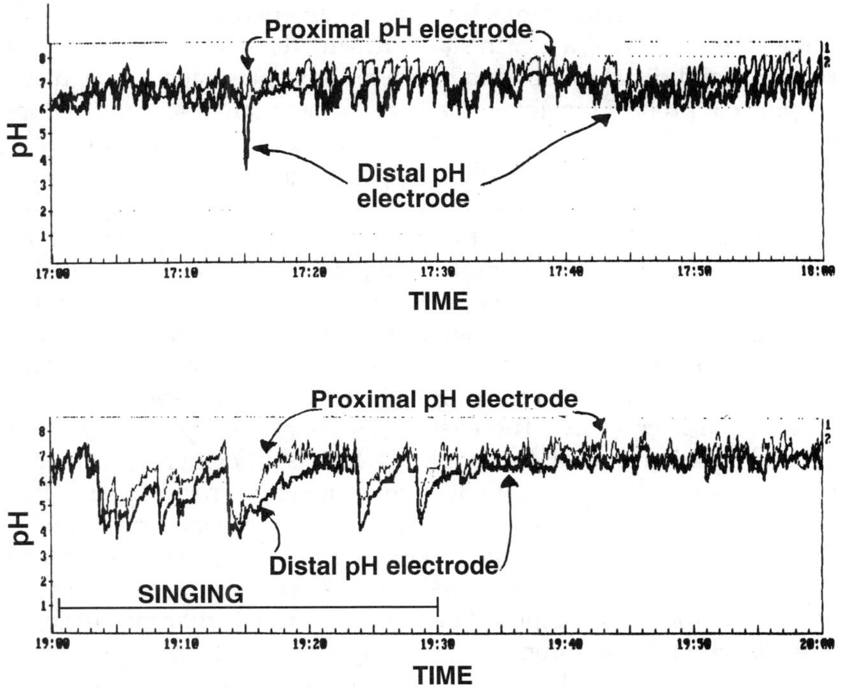

Figure 7–1. Dual-electrode pH probe monitoring in a patient singing for a 30-minute period of the 1 hour shown. The patient experienced typical heartburn, and increased proximal and distal acid exposure was prominent during singing. (From Sataloff RT. *Professonal Voice: The Science and Art of Professional Care*. 3rd ed. San Diego, CA; 2005:618.)

challenged. Pharyngeal probes (versus esophageal probes) have been developed to assess the degree of acid that reaches the pharynx. However, impedance (and acid) probes may be inaccurate when allowed to dry, as may occur in the pharynx, resulting in "pseudoreflux."[46] The yield on hypopharyngeal probes has been demonstrated to be <50% when all artifacts are excluded.[47] Despite this, studies often rely on pH impedance testing to diagnose LPR, or worse, have no objective testing, making data even more difficult to interpret.[48] Monitoring of pH also requires manometry to determine the location of the LES for accurate data. Even a 1-cm discrepancy in placement causes spurious readings.[49] Finally, norms have not been established for pH in the hypopharynx, although the number of drops below pH 4 and the percentage of time below pH 4 are commonly used parameters. Unfortunately, this placement creates difficulty in standardizing the distance between the proximal and distal probes and interferes with placement of the distal esophageal probe 5 cm above the LES, the standard used in developing normal values. Probes in the hypopharynx can be uncomfortable, normal values are not available, and pharyngeal probe data are occasionally subject to interpretation error, including incorrect diagnosis of reflux due to probe drying or to acidic food or liquid ingestion—both artifacts resulting in a drop of pH to <4, which is not a true reflux episode. Some investigators believe that pharyngeal probe placement is important and that data are valid and reliable. Golub and colleagues[50] studied 15 patients with LPR symptoms by a simultaneous standard dual pH probe and a Restech oropharyngeal probe (Respiratory Technology, San Diego, CA). The Restech oropharyngeal probe measures pH and liquid or aerosolized droplets, which is different from standard pH probes, which require a liquid environment for proper functioning. Their data showed that the oropharyngeal probe correlated closely with the sensor near the UES when calculating percentage of time of acid exposure. Wiener et al[51] compared the Restech oropharyngeal probe with 3 traditional pH probes (2 esophageal and 1 pharyngeal) in 15 patients with LPR symptoms. They reported that the Restech probe was sensitive to detecting pH events that originated in the distal esophagus and migrated toward the oropharynx. They reported also that the traditional criterion of pH <4 as an indicator of LPR might not be useful in the oropharynx. The authors suggested that a "significant pH event" might be redefined as a drop of >3.5 standard deviations from baseline pH. Sun et al[52] described their experience using the Restech system, reporting that it proved sensitive for the detection of acid reflux, was minimally invasive, and was well tolerated by patients. Postma[43] places the proximal probe immediately above the cricopharyngeus, posterior to the larynx. This position prevents drying of the probe and reportedly produces valid data. Postma and his associates[43] consider any pharyngeal acid exposure (even 1 episode) to be abnormal. Although placement of the proximal probe (just above the cricopharyngeus or just below it) remains controversial, the need for dual-probe pH monitoring is clear. Without a proximal probe, the sensitivity of single-probe esophageal pH monitoring has been shown to be only 62% for LPR.[44] That is, 38% of patients had pharyngeal reflux with distal esophageal acid exposure parameters that were considered within normal limits. A recent large study by Harrell et al[53] has suggested that there is value in using a hypopharyngeal sensor. Hypopharyngeal sensors are also being studied with pH-impedance equipment (see the section "Role of combined multichannel intraluminal impedance pH" later in this chapter). At present, normal values for distal reflux at 5 cm above the LES and for proximal reflux 20 cm above the sphincter are available, making this a more useful protocol.[54,55] Normal values vary slightly among laboratories, and reference ranges should be included with reports from the laboratory performing the procedure.

The microcomputer (data logger) has a symptom button that allows recording of up to 6 symptoms during a single study. The patient is asked to push the symptom button as well as to record symptoms on a diary card. This dual-entry system allows correlation of reflux events with symptoms in order to determine a symptom index,[56] which is especially valuable in patients with asthma, cough, and chest pain and allows correlation between symptoms and reflux in patients who continue to have symptoms while on medical therapy. Symptom correlation in the otolaryngologic patient may be more difficult on a single study, particularly when symptoms are continuous and not produced by a single reflux episode. This scenario is more likely in patients with laryngitis or chronic sore throat. Other symptoms, such as throat clearing, cough, or those provoked by singing, may be correlated with single reflux episodes.

Prolonged pH monitoring is used in patients with heartburn to establish a diagnosis when symptoms have not responded to a trial of antireflux therapy and endoscopy is negative. In this case, a single-channel pH probe can be placed with the distal probe 5 cm above the LES. Symptoms are correlated with reflux, and reflux frequency is assessed. Patients with known GERD who have heartburn and regurgitation not responding to medical therapy can be monitored while still on therapy with a dual-channel intragastric and distal esophageal probe to assess the adequacy of gastric acid suppression and the frequency of esophageal reflux and to correlate symptoms with reflux events. Patients with continued esophageal acid exposure and/or symptoms may require additional therapy.

Patients with otolaryngologic symptoms or other upper airway symptoms suggestive of GERD are ideal candidates for prolonged ambulatory pH monitoring. We prefer performing monitoring early in the clinical course to establish a diagnosis and to allow symptom correlation when possible. Dual-channel pH monitoring with one electrode 5 cm above the LES and a second probe 20 cm above in the proximal esophagus just below the UES (Figure 7–2) is our procedure of choice. Abnormal distal esophageal acid exposure can be documented, establishing a diagnosis of GERD. Abnormal proximal reflux can be demonstrated, suggesting the potential for aspiration and lending stronger

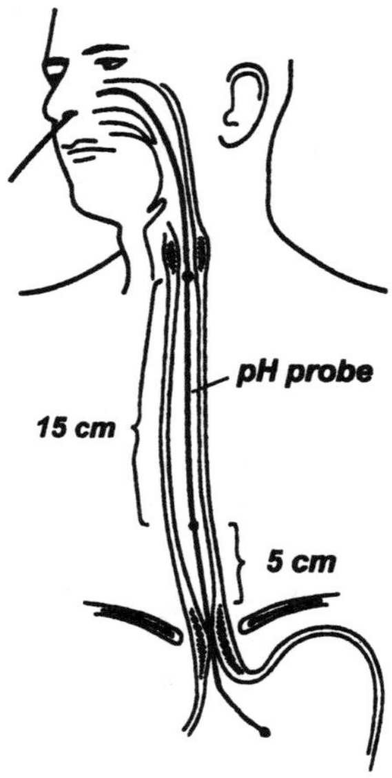

Figure 7–2. Illustration of dual-channel antimony pH probe with electrodes 15 cm apart. Distal electrode is placed 5 cm above the LES. Proximal electrode is 20 cm above the lower sphincter, just below the UES.

probability that the otolaryngologic symptom is due to GERD. If symptom correlation can be demonstrated, this finding will establish the diagnosis. The presence of proximal reflux appears to predict the response to medical therapy in patients with pulmonary disease.[57,58]

This is less clear in the otolaryngologic patient. In a small percentage of patients, percent time of distal esophageal acid exposure will be normal, but an increased frequency of proximal reflux or reflux into the hypopharynx can be demonstrated. This is seen in up to 30% of patients with otolaryngologic symptoms. In one study of 10 patients with reflux laryngitis, 3 of 10 (30%) demonstrated hypopharyngeal reflux with normal distal acid exposure.[57] In a larger, retrospective series of patients with pulmonary disease, 12% of patients had only abnormal proximal reflux,[58] a group that would have been diagnosed incorrectly as normal had only a single-channel study been performed. Reflux in these patients should be considered abnormal and treated aggressively. Studies in our laboratory have shown that dual-electrode pH recording can document abnormal distal and proximal esophageal reflux induced by singing (see Figure 7–1). The singing challenge shown in Figure 7–1 can also unmask significant reflux in patients with otherwise normal 24-hour pH monitoring.

Studies in adults with a variety of otolaryngologic symptoms demonstrate abnormal amounts of acid in reflux in up to 75% of patients.[21] Abnormal acid exposure has been documented in upright and supine positions, although upright reflux seems more common. Ambulatory pH monitoring is most useful in assessing response to antireflux therapy, particularly in the patient who has failed to respond to a therapeutic trial of a proton-pump inhibitor given twice daily for 8 to 12 weeks. Intragastric, distal esophageal, and proximal esophageal pH can be monitored while therapy is continued. Adequacy of intragastric acid suppression can be assessed, as can the presence of esophageal acid exposure and correlation between reflux events and symptoms. This study is particularly valuable in patients who do not respond (or are resistant) to proton-pump inhibitors. If acid reflux is still present, treatment can be increased or modified. If adequate acid suppression is achieved and symptoms persist, an alternative diagnosis can be sought. However, the definition of "adequate acid suppression" is more complex than it might appear. For example, Shi et al[59] reviewed 771 consecutive patients who had undergone 24-hour pH monitoring studies. Statistically significant association was found between symptoms during reflux episodes in 96 patients (12.5%) with esophageal acid exposures that were within the laboratories' normal values. In these patients, the duration of reflux episodes was shorter, and the pH of reflux episodes was higher than in patients who were diagnosed with GERD. The authors hypothesized that the underlying pathologic feature in these patients was hypersensitivity to acid. However, there are other possible explanations—for example, normative values may have been established at levels higher than desirable.

An area of some controversy is the evaluation of the patient with continued symptoms but no esophageal acid exposure on 24-hour pH monitoring. In such cases, the possibility of alkaline or pH-neutral reflux may be raised. Current pH monitoring technology makes it possible to detect bilirubin pigment (bile) by use of a Bilitec probe in addition to standard probes used for 24-hour pH monitoring. However, current data obtained using this technique suggest that esophageal bile reflux rarely, if ever, occurs in the absence of acid reflux, making the Bilitec probe useful only in select patients (see "Approach to the patient with otolaryngologic abnormalities related to GERD" in this chapter).

The diagnosis of alkaline reflux should not be made based solely on the rise in pH above 7; careful analysis of pH rises above 7 coupled with symptom correlation may suggest alkaline reflux, but it is rarely, if ever, diagnosed conclusively by pH testing. A new approach to detecting pH-neutral reflux, under research currently, uses measurements of electrical impedance at numerous points along an esophageal probe. This device detects the presence of liquid in the esophagus regardless of pH, and sequential measurements along the chain of sensors indicate whether the liquid is traveling from proximal to distal or is refluxing from distal to proximal. This technology requires further study but appears promising. However, the decision to proceed with surgical management for the suspicion of alkaline or pH-neutral reflux is a clinical one and must be made after careful consultation among members of the health care team, including the patient. Current pH technology cannot confirm this diagnosis definitely.

Although prolonged pH monitoring is used extensively in the evaluation of patients with suspected LPR, controversy exists as to its overall sensitivity and specificity. This is particularly important when addressing the issue of hypopharyngeal reflux. A recent study by Shaker and colleagues[60] found a similar number and duration of hypopharyngeal reflux events in control subjects and patients with suspected LPR. Another study[61] revealed no major difference between hypopharyngeal acid exposure in 36 patients with LPR signs and symptoms and healthy controls. Using a new methodology for triple-probe monitoring, Maldonado et al[62] found a 10% prevalence of abnormal pH in normal controls. These data remind us of the importance of standardization of the measurement of hypopharyngeal reflux to optimally understand the causal relationship between this phenomenon and LPR.

Sato et al[63] described their experience using a tetra-probe 24-hour pH monitoring system. The proximal probe is placed in the hypopharynx; a second probe is placed in the mid-esophagus; the third probe is placed a few centimeters above the LES (but not specifically 5 cm); and the distal sensor is placed in the stomach. This system is advantageous in that it measures pH simultaneously at all 4 sites, providing information regarding the relationship of these values. However, in our opinion, there are significant disadvantages associated with failure to have a sensor 5 cm above the LES, a standard site that permits comparison with other literature. In a separate report,[64] the authors described their results using the tetra-probe 24-hour pH monitoring system to evaluate patterns of LPR and GERD and to determine the validity of using pH 5.0 as an indicator of LPR. The data suggest that pH levels <4 and <5 are indicative of significant LPR events. An interesting study was reported in 2010 by Zelenik et al.[65] They performed a prospective dual-probe pH monitoring study in 46 patients with complaints of globus pharyngeus for more than 3 months. They collected data from this group using a pH <4 and from a second data group using pH both <4 and <5. Extraesophageal reflux was found in 23.9% of their patients using analysis of pH <4. When data were calculated using pH both <4 and <5, they found extraesophageal reflux in an additional 4 (8.7%) patients whose reflux had not been detected when pH <4 alone was used.

In addition, abnormal findings on pH monitoring do not necessarily predict patient response to therapy. Similarly, a recent placebo-controlled study[66] of 145 patients treated with either esomeprazole or placebo found that symptomatic or laryngeal improvement was independent of pretherapy pH-monitoring results. The apparent dichotomy in the clinical usefulness of hypopharyngeal pH monitoring is likely due to several key factors:

1. Lack of consensus on the duration and amount of reflux that constitutes abnormal pharyngeal acid exposure
2. High operator dependence and variability of probe positioning (eg, use of manometry vs direct visualization)
3. Variable sensitivity of pH monitoring in detecting reflux, which may vary from day to day.[67]

All these variables have been reported to result in a diagnostic yield from 14% to 83%.[68] The yield may improve with better data evaluation parameters. Reichel and Issing[69] suggest the use of reflux area indices of 4 and 5, which would include time at pH 5. The data regarding pepsin activity at pH 5 have generated somewhat less controversy than the data on activity at higher pH. The reflux area index is calculated from the number and duration of proximal reflux events and the degree to which the pH drops below a given value.[69] Incorporating several data points and including a reflux area index of 5 may increase the sensitivity of pH monitoring.

As such, 24-hour pH monitoring cannot be used to conclusively establish or rule out reflux as the cause of suspected LPR. Until the value of other tests such as wireless esophageal pH monitoring and/or impedance monitoring (see later section) has been established, an empiric trial with a proton-pump inhibitor remains the most important determinant of the relationship between reflux and LPR symptoms.

TELEMETRY CAPSULE PH MONITORING

The development of telemetry capsule-based (tubeless) pH monitoring has added to laryngologists' armamentarium and ability to monitor patients with suspected reflux disease. The system is safe, well tolerated, and reliable, allowing 48-hour assessment of esophageal acid exposure. It is unobtrusive, comfortable, and allows longer duration of acid monitoring. Its use in LPR has not been studied, and the technology is limited by current inability to place the capsule proximally due to discomfort and bulk. Further refinements in methodology, recording protocols, and diagnostic accuracy have made this an extremely useful test in typical GERD patients. One of us (P.O.K.) uses the telemetry capsule to perform off-therapy monitoring in patients prior to antireflux surgery to be certain that abnormal acid exposure is present prior to an operation. This new technology will likely become valuable in assessing patients with LPR.[70]

ROLE OF COMBINED MULTICHANNEL INTRALUMINAL IMPEDANCE PH

Combined multichannel intraluminal impedance (MII) and pH monitoring is a promising technique that identifies gas, liquid, and mixed gastroesophageal reflux and allows differentiation of them into acid (pH <4) and nonacid (pH >4) types. The current catheter allows simultaneous monitoring of intragastric and distal esophageal pH with the ability to assess the height of refluxate from 3 to 17 cm above the LES. Early data suggest that a number of patients with so-called extraesophageal disease may have symptoms associated with nonacid reflux, although the clear relationship of this type of reflux to LPR remains to be studied. Wu[71] reported that combining MII and dual-channel pH monitoring increased the diagnostic yield by ~10% compared with combined MII and single-channel pH monitoring systems. Lee and colleagues[72] reported a 2-fold increase in diagnosing reflux in patients with LPR symptoms, using combined dual-channel impedance/pH-metry. Loots et al[73] reported that the addition of MII to standard pH monitoring increased the yield of symptom association in children and infants with confirmed reflux. Combined MII/pH monitoring is a useful tool in evaluating all patients with persistent symptoms of acid-suppressive therapy, particularly those with LPR.[74]

ESOPHAGEAL MANOMETRY

Manometry will establish abnormal LES pressure or esophageal motility and is necessary preoperatively to evaluate contraction amplitude in the esophageal body. A single measurement of LES pressure is rarely low in patients with GERD. In our experience, only 4% of patients with GERD have a low LES pressure.[75] Esophageal motility abnormalities are found more frequently than a low LES pressure. The most common finding appears to be ineffective esophageal motility (IEM) (amplitude of contraction in the distal esophagus <30 mm Hg occurring with 30% or more of water swallows). In our experience, this is the most common abnormality in patients with GERD, seen in ~35% of patients with esophagitis.[75] IEM appears even more commonly in GERD-related laryngitis, asthma, and cough.[76] Esophageal manometry is performed prior to antireflux surgery to be certain that the patient does not have a motility abnormality that would contraindicate surgery (achalasia or scleroderma-like esophagus). Tailoring the operation based on motility findings is likely not necessary; a Nissen fundoplication (360-degree wrap) is likely the best operation in most patients. Patients with IEM and respiratory symptoms do not appear to respond as well to antireflux surgery if respiratory complaints are the presenting symptom.

Esophageal manometry is important also for proper placement of probes for pH monitoring. Although the proximal probe can be positioned accurately by direct vision using a flexible fiber-optic laryngoscope, mirror, or telescope, without manometry there is no way to position the distal probe precisely.[77] However, compared with manometry, even visual proximal probe placement was accurate in only 70% of cases in the study by Johnson et al.[77] Distal probe placement was accurate in just 40% of cases using estimated interprobe distance. Using fixed interprobe distances of 15 cm and 20 cm, distal probe placement was accurate in only 3% and 40%, respectively, of cases. These errors are critical because the normative values for distal esophageal acid exposure were established with the distal probe positioned 5 cm above the LES.[78–81] Even slight modifications in the distance between the distal probe and the LES cause substantial changes in acid exposure data.[82–85]

HIATAL HERNIA

A hiatal hernia is not predictive of reflux as a cause of the patient's symptoms.[86] Up to 60% of patients over the age of 60 years will demonstrate a hiatal hernia identified on barium swallow examination. One study suggested that only 9% of patients with a radiographically demonstrated hernia have typical reflux symptoms.[87]

Hernias do change the relationship of the LES and crural diaphragm. The LES is displaced above the diaphragm. The low pressure in the hernia can act as a reservoir for acid, allowing earlier reflux during LES relaxations, and may delay esophageal clearance.[88] Patients with large hernias who also have low LES pressure may be more prone to reflux[89] if changes occur in intra-abdominal pressure.

EVALUATION FOR THE PRESENCE OF *HELICOBACTER PYLORI*

The bacterium *Helicobacter pylori* appears to play a role in the development of chronic type B gastritis, gastroduodenal ulcer disease, and gastric carcinoma.[90,91] Its significance in GERD remains uncertain, and it is unclear whether treatment for *H. pylori* in reflux patients is necessary or even advisable. *H. pylori* can be detected through serologic determination of immunoglobin G antibodies to the organism. This blood test is performed using an enzyme-linked immunosorbent assay/2-step indirect sandwich assay on directly coated microtiter plates.[92] It is believed to have a sensitivity of 94% and a specificity of 85%.[92]

APPROACH TO THE PATIENT WITH OTOLARYNGOLOGIC ABNORMALITIES RELATED TO GASTROESOPHAGEAL REFLUX DISEASE

In patients with GERD-related otolaryngologic complaints, a detailed history should be obtained, and a thorough physical examination and laryngoscopy should be performed (Figure 7–3). If dysphagia is present, a functional endoscopic evaluation of swallowing or a videoendoscopic swallowing evaluation should be considered, and a barium swallow should be performed to rule out stricture or motility abnormalities. The clinician's dilemma centers on the choice of early diagnostic testing with prolonged pH monitoring or institution of a therapeutic trial of medication. The "best" approach is not clear. Although diagnostic testing with ambulatory pH monitoring would be ideal, there are several limitations: (1) pH monitoring is not always available; (2) sensitivity and specificity are clearly not 100%; (3) patients do not reflux with the same frequency every day; and (4) variability in both distal and proximal esophageal acid exposure time in patients with extraesophageal GERD is common,

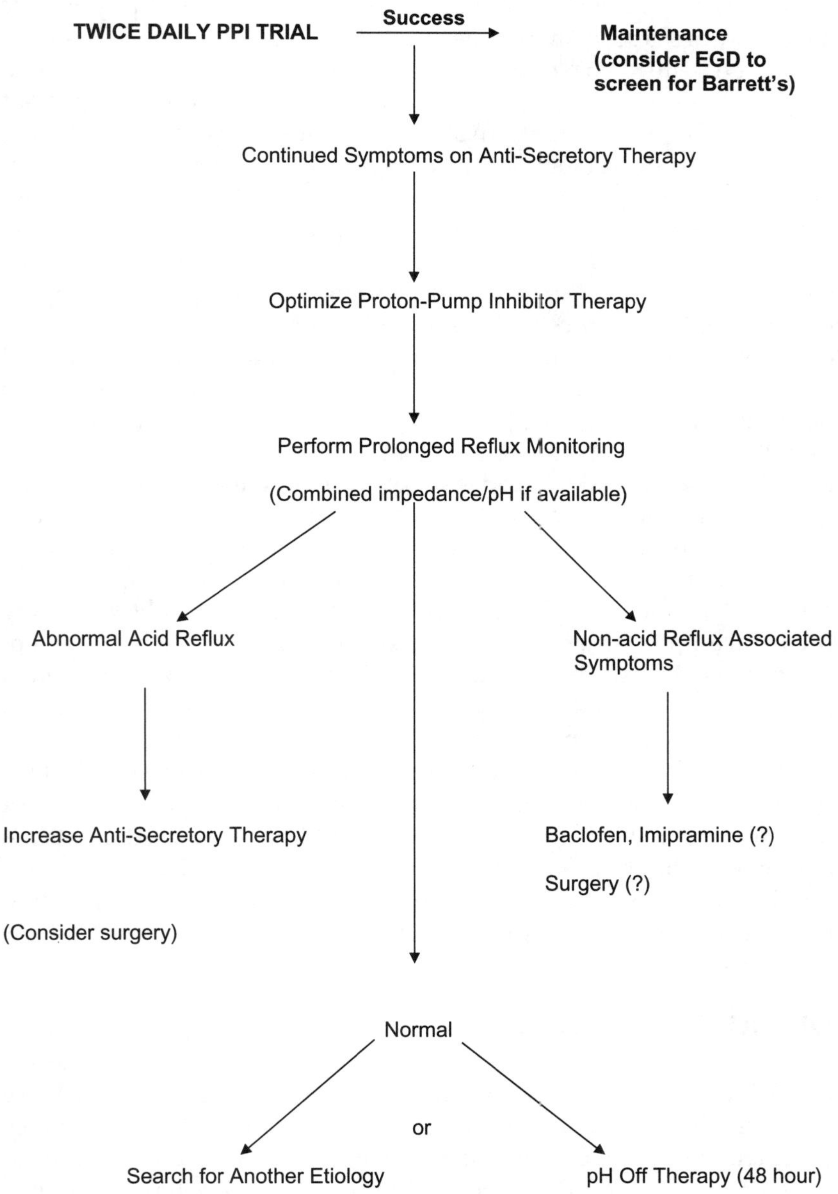

Figure 7–3. Outline of approach to the patient with GERD and otolaryngologic disease. *PPI,* proton-pump inhibitor; *EGD,* esophagogastroduodenoscopy.

increasing the possibility of a false-negative pH study if physiologic acid exposure is seen on a single study.

If the history and findings on laryngoscopic examination raise a high clinical suspicion of GERD or LPR, if prolonged monitoring is not available, if frequent heartburn and regurgitation are present, or if there is endoscopic documentation of GERD or LPR, a therapeutic trial of antireflux therapy is a reasonable initial choice. An early study with empiric omeprazole 40 mg at bedtime in patients with suspected reflux laryngitis found a 67% response in patients with laryngeal symptoms suggestive of GERD.[93] Another study found 70% success with empiric omeprazole 20 mg twice daily for a similar time period.[94] We use a trial of a proton-pump inhibitor twice daily in combination with dietary and behavior modification initially for 8 to 12 weeks. If the patient does not respond, pH monitoring should be performed while proton-pump inhibitor therapy is continued. A dual-channel probe with intragastric and distal esophageal electrodes should be placed to ascertain adequate gastric acid suppression and to assess for presence of esophageal acid exposure. Distal esophageal acid exposure for more than 1.2% of the time is definitely abnormal, and additional medical therapy is indicated.[95] "Normal" esophageal acid exposure, particularly when any proximal esophageal acid exposure is documented, may not always represent a negative study. A positive symptom index may be seen even in patients with "normal" distal acid exposure; and this, too, is abnormal and warrants additional therapy. The *absence* of any esophageal acid exposure and presence of adequate gastric acid suppression (pH >4 for 50% of total monitoring time) suggest adequate medical therapy in most patients, and an alternative diagnosis should be considered. If GERD-associated otolaryngologic disease is documented, endoscopy is indicated in many cases to rule out Barrett's esophagus prior to initiating long-term medical therapy or surgery.

OUTCOME MEASURES

In addition to using instruments discussed elsewhere (such as the Voice Handicap Index[96]) that were designed to measure outcomes of voice disorders, Belafsky and coworkers[97] have introduced the reflux finding score (RFS). The RFS depends on observations of subglottic edema, ventricular obliteration, erythema/hyperemia, vocal fold edema, diffuse laryngeal edema, posterior laryngeal hypertrophy, granuloma/granulation tissue, and thick endolaryngeal mucus. Although additional research from other centers is needed to confirm the validity and reliability of the RFS, the authors found excellent inter- and intraobserver reproducibility (although all observers were practicing at the same medical center); they found the RFS to be an accurate instrument for documenting treatment efficacy in patients with LPR. Other quality-of-life evolutions have highlighted the impact of GERD and LPR on patient function.[98,99]

The Pharyngeal Reflux Symptom Questionnaire was developed by Andersson et al.[100] It is a self-administered questionnaire specific for LPR patients. They compared this tool with the LPR–Health Related Quality of Life and the reflux symptom index and reported strong correlation. The authors also reported that the questionnaire discriminated between patients without and with LPR. Several reports[101,102] have suggested that anxiety, depression, and depressive symptoms can impact subjective responses to quality-of-life tools and symptom indices and thus diminish the predictive value of symptom assessment, which raises concern about the usefulness of these tools. Researchers in China[103] reported significantly higher Voice Handicap Index scores and higher depression scores in their patients with LPR. Nishimura et al[104] evaluated postoperative LPR in patients who had undergone surgery for esophageal cancer. They proposed a classification system for grading findings on endoscopy to facilitate more accurate diagnosis of LPR in this patient population.

REFERENCES

1. Bough ID, Castell DO, Sataloff RT, Hills JR. Gastroesophageal reflux laryngitis resistant to omeprazole therapy. *J Voice.* 1995;9:205–211.
2. Klinkenberg-Knoll EC, Meuwissen GSM. Combined gastric and oesophageal 24-hour pH monitoring and oesophageal manometry in patients with reflux disease, resistant to treatment with omeprazole. *Aliment Pharmacol Ther.* 1990;4:485–495.
3. Kotby MN, Hassan O, El-Makhzangy AM, Farahat M, Milad P. Gastroesophageal reflux/laryngopharyngeal reflux disease: a critical analysis of the literature. *Eur Arch Otorhinolaryngol.* 2010;267: 171–179.
4. Ayazi S, Hagen JA, Zehetner J, et al. Loss of alkalization in proximal esophagus: a new diagnostic paradigm for patients with laryngopharyngeal reflux. *J Gastrointest Surg.* 2010;14:1653–1659.

5. Chong VH. Laryngopharyngeal reflux is not always secondary to gastroesophageal reflux. *Eur Arch Otolaryngol.* 2010;267:321–322.

6. Chong VH. Examination of the aero-digestive tract during routine endoscopy. *Dig Liver Dis.* 2010;42:74.

7. Ott DJ, Wu WC, Gelfand DW. Reflux esophagitis revisited: prospective analysis of radiologic accuracy. *Gastrointest Radiol.* 1981;6:1–7.

8. Richter JE, Castell DO. Gastroesophageal reflux: pathogenesis, diagnosis, and therapy. *Ann Intern Med.* 1982;97:93–103.

9. Ott DJ. Gastroesophageal reflux: what is the role of barium studies? *AJR Am J Roentgenol.* 1994;162:627–629.

10. Thompson JK, Koehler RE, Richter JE. Detection of gastroesophageal reflux: value of barium studies compared with 24-hour pH monitoring. *AJR.* 1994;162:621–626.

11. Koufman JA, Amin MR, Panetti M. Prevalence of reflux in 113 consecutive patients with laryngeal and voice disorders. *Otolaryngol Head Neck Surg.* 2000;123:385–388.

12. Sellar RJ, DeCaestecker JS, Heading RC. Barium radiology: a sensitive test for gastro-oesophageal reflux. *Clin Radiol.* 1987;38:303–307.

13. Malmud LS, Fisher RS. Radionuclide studies of esophageal transit and gastroesophageal reflux. *Sem Nucl Med.* 1982;12:104–114.

14. Jenkins AF, Cowan RJ, Richter JE. Gastroesophageal scintigraphy: is it a sensitive test for gastroesophageal reflux disease? *J Clin Gastroenterol.* 1985;7:127–131.

15. Hetzel DJ, Dent J, Reed WD, et al. Healing and relapse of some peptic esophagitis after treatment with omeprazole. *Gastroenterology.* 1988;95:903–912.

16. Winters C Jr, Spurling TJ, Chobanian SJ, et al. Barrett's esophagus: a prevalent, occult complication of gastroesophageal reflux disease. *Gastroenterology.* 1987;92:118–124.

17. Lieberman DA, Oehlke M, Helfand M. Risk factors for Barrett's esophagus in community based practice. *Am J Gastroenterol.* 1997;92:1293–1297.

18. Cherian P, Smith LF, Bardham KD, Thorpe J, Oakley GD, Dawson D. Esophageal tests in the evaluation of non-cardiac chest pain. *Dis Esophagus.* 1995;8:129–133.

19. Harding SM, Guzzo MR, Richter JE. Prevalence of GERD in asthmatics without reflux symptoms. *Gastroenterology.* 1997;4:A141.

20. Sontag SJ, O'Connell S, Khandelwal S, et al. Most asthmatics have gastroesophageal reflux with or without bronchodilator therapy. *Gastroenterology.* 1990;99:613–618.

21. Wiener GJ, Koufman JA, Wu WC, et al. Chronic hoarseness secondary to gastroesophageal reflux disease. *Am J Gastroenterol.* 1989;84:503–508.

22. Katsinelos P, Kountouras J, Chatzimavroudis G, et al. Should inspection of the laryngopharyngeal area be part of routine upper gastrointestinal endoscopy? A prospective study. *Dig Liver Dis.* 2009;41:283–288.

23. DeVault KR, Castell DO. Guidelines for the diagnosis and treatment of gastroesophageal reflux disease. *Arch Intern Med.* 1995;155:2165–2173.

24. Hetzel DJ, Dent J, Reed WO, et al. Healing and relapse of severe peptic esophagitis after treatment with omeprazole. *Gastroenterology.* 1988;95:903–912.

25. Eller R, Ginsburg M, Lurie D, Heman-Ackah YD, Lyons KM, Sataloff RT. Flexible laryngoscopy: a comparison of fiber optic and distal chip technologies—part 2: laryngopharyngeal reflux. *J Voice.* 2009;23:389–395.

26. Gawron A, Hirano I. Advances in diagnostic testing for gastroesophageal reflux disease. *World J Gastroenterol.* 2010;16:3750–3756.

27. Tseng PH, Chen CC, Chiu HM, et al. Performance of narrow band imaging and magnification endoscopy in the prediction of therapeutic response in patients with gastroesophageal reflux disease. *J Clin Gastroenterol.* 2011;45:501–506.

28. Gaddam S, Sharma P. Advances in endoscopic diagnosis and treatment of Barrett's esophagus. *J Dig Dis.* 2010;11:323–333.

29. Mannath J, Ragunath K. Era of Barrett's surveillance: does equipment matter? *World J Gastroenterol.* 2010;16:4640–4645.

30. Goetz M, Kiesslich R. Advanced imaging of the gastrointestinal tract: research vs. clinical tools? *Curr Opin Gastroenterol.* 2009;25:412–421.

31. Hoffman A, Basting N, Goetz M, et al. High-definition endoscopy with i-Scan and Lugol's solution for more precise detection of mucosal breaks in patients with reflux symptoms. *Endoscopy*. 2009;41:107–112.

32. Kawahara Y, Okada H, Kawano S, et al. New digital imaging technology i-Scan for upper GI endoscopy: a pilot study. *Gastrointest Endosc*. 2009;69:AB377.

33. Hoffman A, Sar F, Goetz M, et al. High definition colonoscopy combined with iScan is superior in the detection of colorectal neoplasias compared with standard video colonoscopy: a prospective randomized controlled trial. *Endoscopy*. 2010;42:827–833.

34. Hoffman A, Kagel C, Goetz M, et al. Recognition and characterization of small colonic neoplasia with high-definition colonoscopy using iScan is as precise as chromoendoscopy. *Dig Liver Dis*. 2010;42:45–50.

35. Mannath J, Ragunath K. Era of Barrett's surveillance: does equipment matter? *World J Gastroenterol*. 2010;16:4640–4645.

36. Boudoux C, Leuin S, Oh WY, et al. Optical microscopy of the pediatric vocal fold. *Arch Otolaryngol HNS*. 2009;13:53–64.

37. Chang EW, Kobler JB, Yun SH. Triggered optical coherence tomography for capturing rapid periodic motion. *Sci Rep*. 2011;1:1–7.

38. Suter MJ, Vakoc BJ, Yachimski PS, et al. Comprehensive microscopy of the esophagus in human patients with optical frequency domain imaging. *Gastrointest Endosc*. 2008;68:745–753.

39. Kang DK, Suter MJ, Boudoux C, et al. Comprehensive imaging of gastroesophageal biopsy samples by spectrally encoded confocal microscopy. *Gastrointest Endosc*. 2010;71:35–43.

40. Ismail-Beigi F, Horton PF, Pope CE. Histological consequences of gastroesophageal reflux in man. *Gastroenterology*. 1970;58:163–174.

41. Winter CS, Madara JL, Stafford RJ. Intraepithelial eosinophils: a new diagnostic criterion for reflux esophagitis. *Gastroenterology*. 1982;83:818–823.

42. Falk GW. Barrett's esophagus. In: Castell DO, Richter JE, eds. *The Esophagus*. Malden, MA: Wiley-Blackwell; 2012:509–539.

43. Postma GN. Ambulatory pH monitoring methodology. *Ann Otol Rhinol Laryngol Suppl*. 2000;184:10–14.

44. Postma GN, Belafsky PC, Aviv JE, Koufman JA. Laryngopharyngeal reflux testing. *Ear Nose Throat J*. 2002;81(9 Suppl):14–18.
45. Muderris T, Gokcan MK, Yorulmaz I. The clinical value of pharyngeal pH monitoring using a double-probe, triple-sensor catheter. *Arch Otolaryngol HNS*. 2009;135:163–167.
46. Wiener GJ, Koufman JA, Wu WC, et al. Chronic hoarseness secondary to gastroesophageal reflux disease: documentation with 24-h ambulatory pH monitoring. *Am J Gastroenterol*. 1989;84:1503–1508.
47. Harrell SP, Koopman J, Woosley S, et al. Exclusion of pH artifacts is essential for hypopharyngeal pH monitoring. *Laryngoscope*. 2007;117:470–474.
48. Joniau S, Bradshaw A, Esterman A, et al. Reflux and laryngitis: a systematic review. *Otolaryngol Head Neck Surg*. 2007;136:686–692.
49. Postma GN, Belafsky PC, Aviv JE, et al. Laryngopharyngeal reflux testing. *Ear Nose Throat J*. 2002;81(9 suppl 2):14–18.
50. Golub JS, Johns MM 3rd, Lim JH, Del Gaudio JM, Klein AM. Comparison of an oropharyngeal pH probe and a standard dual pH probe for diagnosis of laryngopharyngeal reflux. *Ann Otol Rhinol Laryngol*. 2009;118:1–5.
51. Wiener G, Tsukashima R, Kelly C, et al. Oropharyngeal pH monitoring for the detection of liquid and aerosolized supraesophageal gastric reflux. *J Voice*. 2009;101:498–504.
52. Sun G, Muddana S, Slaugther JC, et al. A new pH catheter for laryngopharyngeal reflux: normal values. *Laryngoscope*. 2009;119:1639–1643.
53. Harrell S, Evans B, Goudy S, et al. Design and implementation of an ambulatory pH monitoring protocol in patients with suspected laryngopharyngeal reflux. *Laryngoscope*. 2005;115:89–92.
54. Katz PO. Ambulatory esophageal and hypopharyngeal pH monitoring in patients with hoarseness. *Am J Gastroenterol*. 1990;85:38.
55. Johnson LF, DeMeester TR. Twenty-four hour pH monitoring of the distal esophagus. *Am J Gastroenterol*. 1974;62:325–333.
56. Wiener GJ, Richter JE, Copper PA, Wu WC, Castell DO. The symptom index: a clinically important parameter of ambulatory 24-hour esophageal pH monitoring. *Am J Gastroenterol*. 1988;83:358–361.

57. Dobhan R, Castell DO. Normal and abnormal proximal esophageal acid exposure: results of ambulatory dual-probe pH monitoring. *Am J Gastroenterol.* 1993;88:25–29.

58. Schnatz PF, Castell JA, Castell DO. Pulmonary symptoms associated with gastroesophageal reflux: use of ambulatory pH monitoring to diagnose and to direct therapy. *Am J Gastroenterol.* 1996;91:1715–1718.

59. Shi G, des Varannes SB, Scarpignato C, Le Rhun M, Galmiche JP. Reflux related symptoms in patients with normal oesophageal exposure to acid. *Gut.* 1995;37:457–464.

60. Shaker R, Bardan E, Gu C, et al. Intrapharyngeal distribution of gastric acid refluxate. *Laryngoscope.* 2003;113:1182–1191.

61. Bilgen C, Ogut F, Kesimli-Dinc H, et al. The comparison of an empiric proton pump inhibitor trial vs 24-hour double-probe pH monitoring in laryngopharyngeal reflux. *J Laryngol Otol.* 2003;117:386–390.

62. Maldonado A, Diederich L, Castell D, et al. Laryngopharyngeal reflux identified using a new catheter design: defining normal values and excluding artifacts. *Laryngoscope.* 2003;113:349–355.

63. Sato K, Umeno H, Chitose S, Nakashima T. Tetra-probe, 24-hour pH monitoring for laryngopharyngeal reflux: a technique for simultaneous study of hypopharynx, esophagus and stomach. *J Laryngol Otol.* 2009;123(suppl 31):117–122.

64. Sato K, Umeno H, Chitose S, Nakashima T. Patterns of laryngopharyngeal and gastroesophageal reflux. *J Laryngol Otol.* 2009;123(suppl 31):42–47.

65. Zelenik K, Matousek P, Urban O, Schwarz P, Starek I, Kominek P. Globus pharyngeus and extraesophageal reflux: simultaneous pH <4.0 and pH <5.0 analysis. *Laryngoscope.* 2010;120:2160–2164.

66. Vaezi MF, Richter J, Stasney CR, et al. A randomized double-blind placebo controlled study of acid suppression for the treatment of suspected laryngopharyngeal reflux. *Gastroenterology.* 2004;126:A40.

67. Ulualp SO, Toohill RJ, Shaker R, et al. Outcomes of acid suppressive therapy in patients with posterior laryngitis. *Otolaryngol Head Neck Surg.* 2001;124:16–22.

68. El-Sayed Ali M. Laryngopharyngeal reflux: diagnosis and treatment of a controversial disease. *Curr Opin Allergy Clin Immunol.* 2008;8:28–33.

69. Reichel O, Issing WJ. Impact of different pH thresholds for 24-h dual probe pH monitoring in patients with suspected laryngopharyngeal reflux. *J Laryngol Otol.* 2008;122:485–489.

70. Pandolfino JE, Kahrilas PJ. Prolonged pH monitoring: Bravo capsule. *GI Clin North Am.* 2005;15:307–318.

71. Wu JCY. Combined multichannel intraluminal impedance and pH monitoring for patients with suspected laryngopharyngeal reflux: is it ready to use? *J Neurogastroenterol Motil.* 2010;16:108–109.

72. Lee BE, Kim GH, Ryu DY, et al. Combined dual channel impedance/pH-metry in patients with suspected laryngopharyngeal reflux. *J Neurogastroenterol Motil.* 2010;16:157–165.

73. Loots CM, Benninga MA, Davidson GP, Omari TI. Addition of pH-impedance monitoring (pH-MII) to standard pH monitoring increases the yield of symptom association analysis in infants and children with gastroesophageal reflux. *J Pediatr.* 2009;154:248–252.

74. Tutuian R, Castell DO. Reflux monitoring: role of combined multichannel intraluminal impedance and pH. *GI Clin North Am.* 2005; 15:361–371.

75. Barrett J, Peghini P, Katz P, Castell J, Castell D. Ineffective esophageal motility (IEM): the most common manometric abnormality in GERD. *Gastroenterology.* 1997;112. Abstract 66.

76. Harding SM, Richter JE, Guzzo MR, et al. Asthma and gastroesophageal reflux: acid suppressive therapy improves asthma outcome. *Am J Med.* 1996;100:395–405.

77. Johnson PE, Koufman JA, Nowak LJ, Belafsky PC, Postma GN. Ambulatory 24-hour double-probe pH monitoring: the importance of manometry. *Laryngoscope.* 2001;111:1970–1975.

78. Johnson LF, DeMeester TR. Twenty-four hour pH monitoring of the distal esophagus. *Am J Gastroenterol.* 1974;62:325–332.

79. Rosen S, Pope C III. Extended esophageal pH monitoring. An analysis of the literature and assessment of its role in the diagnosis and management of gastroesophageal reflux. *J Clin Gastroenterol.* 1989;11:260–270.

80. Mattox HE III, Richter JE. Prolonged ambulatory esophageal pH monitoring in the evaluation of gastroesophageal reflux disease. *Am J Med.* 1990;89:345–356.

81. Richter JE, Bradley LA, DeMeester TR, Wu WC. Normal 24-hour ambulatory esophageal pH values: influence of study center, pH electrode, age, and gender. *Dig Dis Sci.* 1992;37:849–856.

82. Johansson KE, Tibbling L. Gastric secretion and reflux pattern in reflux oesophagitis before and during ranitidine treatment. *Scand J Gastroenterol.* 1986;21:487–492.

83. Haase GM, Ross MN, Gance-Cleveland B, Kolack KE. Extended four-channel esophageal pH monitoring: the importance of acid reflux patterns at the middle and proximal levels. *J Pediatr Surg.* 1988;23(1 pt 2):32–37.

84. Lehamn G, Rogers D, Cravens E, Flueckiger J. Prolonged pH probe testing less than 5 cm above the lower esophageal sphincter (LES): establishing normal control values. *Gastroenterology.* 1990;98:77.

85. Weusten BL, Akkermans LM, Van Berge-Henegouwen GP, Smout AJ. Spatiotemporal characteristics of physiological gastroesophageal reflux. *Am J Physiol.* 1994;266(3 pt 1):G357–G362.

86. Sloan S, Rademaker AW, Kahrilas PJ. Determinants of gastroesophageal junction incompetence: hiatal hernia, lower esophageal sphincter, or both? *Ann Intern Med.* 1992;117:977–982.

87. Fouad YM, Koury R, Hatlebakk JG, Katz PO, Castell DO. Ineffective esophageal motility (IEM) is more prevalent in reflux patients with respiratory symptoms. *Gastroenterology.* 1998;114. Abstract 6506.

88. Palmer ED. The hiatus-esophagitis-esophageal stricture complex. Twenty-year prospective study. *Am J Med.* 1968;44:566–572.

89. Sloan S, Kakrilas PJ. Impairment of esophageal emptying with hiatal hernia. *Gastroenterology.* 1991;100:596–605.

90. NIH Consensus Conference. *Helicobacter pylori* in peptic ulcer disease. NIH Consensus Development Panel on *Helicobacter pylori* in Peptic Ulcer Disease. *JAMA.* 1994;272:65–69.

91. World Health Organization. Schistosomes, liver flukes and *Helicobacter pylori. IARC Monogr Eval Carcinog Risks Hum.* 1994;61:177–220.

92. Nilius M, Malfertheiner P. Diagnostic Procedures for Helicobacter Pylori Infection. In: Malfertheiner P, Hrsg. *Helicobacter pylori: Basis for Therapy.* Stuttgart, Germany: George Thieme-Verlag; 1996.

93. Wo JM, Grist WJ, Gussack G, Delguadio JM, Waring JP. Empiric trial of high-dose omeprazole in patients with posterior laryngitis: a prospective study. *Am J Gastroenterol.* 1997;92:2160–2165.

94. Metz DC, Childs ML, Ruiz C, Weinstein GS. Pilot study of the oral omeprazole test for reflux laryngitis. *Otolaryngol Head Neck Surg.* 1997;116:41–46.

95. Kuo B, Castell DO. Optimal dosing of omeprazole 40 mg daily: effects on gastric and esophageal pH and serum gastrin in healthy controls. *Am J Gastroenterol.* 1996;91:1532–1538.

96. Jacobson BH, Johnson A, Grywalski C, et al. The Voice Handicap Index (VHI): development and validation. *Am J Speech-Lang Pathol.*1997;6:66–70.

97. Belafsky PC, Postma GN, Koufman JA. The validity and reliability of the reflux finding score. *Laryngoscope.* 2001;111:1313–1317.

98. Rivicki DA, Wood M, Maton PN, et al. The impact of gastroesophageal reflux disease on health-related quality of life. *Am J Med.* 1998;104:252–258.

99. Lenderking WR, Hillson E, Rawler C, et al. The clinical characteristics and impact of laryngopharyngeal reflux disease on health-related quality of life. *Value Health.* 2003;6:560–565.

100. Andersson O, Rydén A, Ruth M, Möller RY, Finizia C. Development and validation of a laryngopharyngeal reflux questionnaire, the Pharyngeal Reflux Symptoms Questionnaire. *Scand J Gastroenterol.* 2010;45:147–159.

101. Oyer SL, Anderson LC, Halum SL. Influence of anxiety and depression on the predictive value of the Reflux Symptom Index. *Ann Otol Rhinol Laryngol.* 2009;118:687–692.

102. Elam JC, Ishman SL, Dunbar KB, Clarke JO, Gourin CG. The relationship between depressive symptoms and Voice Handicap Index scores in laryngopharyngeal reflux. *Laryngoscope.* 2010;120: 1900–1903.

103. Cheung TK, Lam PK, Wei WI, et al. Quality of life in patients with laryngopharyngeal reflux. *Digestion.* 2009;79:52–57.

104. Nishimura K, Fujita H, Tanaka Y, et al. Endoscopic classification for reflux pharyngolaryngitis. *Dis Esophagus.* 2010;23:20–26.

8

Behavioral and Medical Management of Gastroesophageal Reflux Disease

Gastroesophageal reflux disease (GERD) is a chronic relapsing condition with a variety of symptom presentations caused by the reflux of gastric contents—principally acid and pepsin—into the esophagus or above. Management of the patient with GERD requires careful consideration of the primary symptom presentation, the degree of mucosal injury, and the presence or absence of complications. Treatment focuses on 4 goals: elimination of symptoms, healing of mucosal injury if present, management of complications, and maintenance of symptomatic remission. Treatment should combine lifestyle modifications, pharmacologic therapy, and appropriate use of antireflux surgery. GERD is a chronic condition that may recur quickly if therapy is stopped or medication dosage is decreased; therefore, long-term therapy is the key to effective management and often requires continuous full-prescription doses of appropriate medications. Symptom relief and mucosal healing in GERD are directly related to control of intragastric acid secretion (to limit the time during which gastric pH is <4) and reduction of esophageal acid exposure.[1] Clinical trials in patients with symptomatic erosive esophagitis suggest that a careful and systematic stepwise approach to medical therapy will result in satisfactory symptom relief in more than 90% of patients.[1]

In contrast, there have been relatively few clinical trials of treatment involving patients with asthma, cough, laryngopharyngeal reflux (LPR), and other extraesophageal manifestations of GERD. Most studies have been uncontrolled, and maintenance trials are lacking. Treatment is based on the principles of treatment of heartburn and erosive esophagitis, and on observations from available clinical trials and clinical experience. As a general rule, patients with LPR and the other extraesophageal manifestations of GERD require higher doses of pharmacologic therapy, usually with proton-pump inhibitors (PPIs) twice daily, with longer periods of treatment needed to achieve complete relief of symptoms compared with regimens used in patients with heartburn and erosive esophagitis. Although relief of symptoms, healing of mucosal injury, and maintenance of remission are still the primary goals, assessing these end points is somewhat difficult, as the gold standard for diagnosis is not always clear. This chapter reviews the principles of the medical treatment of GERD, with specific emphasis on LPR and other extraesophageal manifestations of GERD.

LIFESTYLE MODIFICATION AND PATIENT EDUCATION

Simple and effective changes in lifestyle are essential in controlling symptoms of GERD. Educating patients about the recurring nature and chronicity of GERD and LPR is crucial to compliance with long-term medical management. Studies with overnight pH monitoring have shown a significant decrease in total esophageal acid exposure after elevation of the head of the bed 6 inches from exposure incurred while sleeping flat.[2] A similar effect can be produced by placing a foam rubber wedge under the patient's mattress. A long (full-length) wedge is preferable, to tilt the whole mattress rather than bending it at the patient's waist level. An effective alternative approach is to instruct the patient to sleep preferentially lying on the left side. This sleeping posture places the esophagogastric junction in an advantageous position above the gastric contents and has been shown to significantly decrease recumbent reflux.[3]

Elimination of gastric irritants from the diet, or decreasing their intake, may reduce symptoms. Such agents include citrus juices, tomato products, coffee (both caffeinated and decaffeinated), and alcohol. Cola drinks, tea, and other acidic fluids are often overlooked as potential gastric and esophageal irritants.[4] A meal high in fat increases postprandial reflux episodes in patients with GERD,[5] so a low-fat diet is recommended. Chocolate and other carminatives decrease lower esophageal sphincter (LES) pressure, with a corresponding increase in reflux frequency,[6] as do onions, and their intake should be reduced according to most reviews (Table 8–1). Koufman[7] evaluated the clinical impact of a low-acid diet on therapeutic outcome in patients treated for LPR. She studied a group of 20 patients with persistent signs and symptoms of LPR despite twice-daily use of a PPI and a histamine-2 (H_2) blocker at bedtime. The low-acid diet described by Dr Koufman eliminated all foods and beverages with a pH <5. The patients were placed on this diet for a minimum of 2 weeks, and both the reflux symptom index and the reflux finding score were determined before and after the diet. Koufman's findings show that both the clinical signs and symptoms in these patients with persistent symptoms despite PPI treatment improved following an acid-free diet.

Gastric distention provides the major stimulus for transient LES relaxation, the most common abnormality responsible for individual reflux episodes.[8] Eating large, high-fat meals increases gastric distention and slows gastric emptying, probably increasing transient LES relaxation. Going to sleep on a full stomach or lying down after a meal also creates a stimulus for transient LES relaxation and is likely to increase reflux. It is therefore critical to remind patients to avoid eating within 2 to 3 hours of sleep and to avoid recumbency after a meal.

Chewing gum, particularly bicarbonate gum, after meals also may reduce reflux symptoms, although the mechanism is not understood

Table 8-1. Lifestyle Modifications for Treatment of Gastroesophageal Reflux

Elevation of head of bed (6 inches)—avoid waterbed

Dietary modifications
1. Lower fat, higher protein
2. Avoid specific irritants
   a. citrus juices
   b. tomato products
   c. coffee, tea
   d. alcohol
   e. colas
   f. onions
3. No eating prior to sleeping (allow at least 2 hours)
4. Avoid chocolate, carminatives (which reduce LES pressure)

Decrease or stop smoking

Avoid potentially harmful medications
1. Affect LES pressure
   a. Anticholinergics
   b. Sedatives/tranquilizers
   c. Theophylline
   d. Prostaglandins
   e. Calcium channel-blockers
2. Potentially cause esophageal injury
   a. Potassium tablets
   b. Ferrous sulfate
   c. Antibiotics (gelatin capsules), eg, tetracycline
   d. NSAIDS, aspirin
   e. Alendronate

LES = Lower esophageal sphincter; NSAIDS = nonsteroidal anti-inflammatory drugs.

fully. Smoak and Koufman[9] studied the effects of chewing regular sugarless gum or sugarless gum containing bicarbonate on pharyngeal and esophageal pH. They demonstrated significant increases in mean pharyngeal and esophageal pH for both types of gum, but the improvements were more pronounced with sugarless gum containing bicarbonate. The beneficial effects of chewing gum lasted twice as long as the actual gum-chewing periods (25 min vs 49 minutes); and the beneficial effects of gum chewing were significantly greater than the buffering effect (in control subjects) obtained by eating a meal. In some patients, gum chewing completely abolished reflux episodes on 24-hour pH monitor study. Additional study is needed, but it appears as if gum chewing may be useful adjunctive antireflux therapy.[9]

Medications that decrease esophageal pressures and promote reflux include anticholinergics, sedatives or tranquilizers, tricyclic antidepressants, theophylline, nitrates, and calcium channel–blocking agents.[10] Many other drugs are known to cause direct esophageal injury (pill-induced esophagitis). The most common are potassium chloride tablets, iron sulfate, gelatin capsule antibiotics, nonsteroidal anti-inflammatory drugs,[10] and alendronate (Fosamax).[11] These agents should be used with caution in patients with GERD. Although there is no direct evidence that these agents cause GERD, they can cause esophageal injury and may make mucosal injury from reflux more severe (see Table 8–1). The effects of these agents vary from patient to patient. Experience suggests that none of these drugs greatly exacerbates GERD, so discontinuing a needed agent is usually not necessary, especially with concomitant use of PPIs.

Smoking may decrease LES pressure and delay esophageal clearance, increasing reflux frequency and potentially worsening mucosal injury. The smoking-related changes are probably due to the effects of nicotine. Smoking may decrease the effectiveness of H_2-receptor antagonists, especially at night (when reflux injury is more severe owing to delayed esophageal clearance of refluxate); however, the effect of smoking on the action of PPIs is not known. Clearly, smoking can be detrimental to overall health—exacerbation of GERD is no exception.

One study examined the effects of lifestyle modifications, including raising the head of the bed 6 inches, eliminating meals before bedtime, and using antacids in the management of patients with respiratory symptoms associated with GERD. Outcomes were compared with those noted in patients not using antireflux measures for 2-month periods. In this study, both esophageal and respiratory symptoms were reported to abate with lifestyle modifications compared with patients not practicing lifestyle modifications. However, no objective changes were noted in pulmonary function, and endoscopy was not performed.[12] This suggests that the addition of the conservative measures outlined in Table 8–1 is useful in treatment of extraesophageal GERD. No studies have specifically examined lifestyle modifications in patients with LPR. However, we routinely recommend the use of these conservative measures, as patients often experience reflux during the postprandial period, even when they are upright.[13]

The importance of including lifestyle modifications as part of a treatment program at a time when very efficacious pharmacologic agents, such as PPIs, are available has been debated. All clinical trials have included these lifestyle changes as part of treatment, so the effect of eliminating them is not known. These lifestyle modifications are easy to explain and implement and are of low economic cost. On the basis of symptom severity and control, patients can decide for themselves how diligent they should be. Some patients with mild, infrequent symptoms may avoid the need for regular prescription medications by following these modifications as recommended. They appear somewhat less likely to be sufficient in many voice professionals, especially singers who experience upright reflux when they sing owing to increased intra-abdominal pressure that occurs with proper voice support. However, if 24-hour pH monitoring studies show that these patients do not experience supine or nocturnal reflux, it may be unnecessary for them to elevate the head of the bed. Head-of-bed elevation can be a substantial inconvenience for performers, who may spend 200 nights or more per year in hotel rooms. Therapies for such patients should be rational and individualized on the basis of symptoms and signs and test results.

OVER-THE-COUNTER AGENTS

Numerous antacids and over-the-counter H_2-receptor antagonists are available for the treatment of symptomatic reflux. These agents should be used exclusively to treat symptoms, such as heartburn that is intermittent, and as adjuncts to prescription therapy for breakthrough symptoms. Symptom relief is similar with equipotent antacids and with all the H_2 antagonists available over the counter. Because patients with LPR often require long-term (or lifetime) therapy with high doses of PPIs or H_2 blockers in full prescription doses, management with over-the-counter (low-dose) H_2 blockers is rarely adequate.

The use of antacids remains controversial. Gaviscon Advance, a liquid alginate suspension that helps prevent reflux by creating a physical antireflux barrier of sodium alginate, also has been shown to be efficacious.[14] Experts agree that these agents should be superfluous if sufficient doses of acid-suppressing medications are used. However, opinions differ regarding the level of control achieved in most patients on the customary doses of PPIs (omeprazole 40 mg daily or the equivalent, now available over the counter) and regarding the importance of occasional episodes of breakthrough reflux. It is well known that reflux may still occur with daily 40-mg doses of omeprazole or with 60-mg doses of lansoprazole (also available over the counter). The occurrence of such episodes has been confirmed by pH monitoring studies, often in clinical settings, and some patients require higher doses for complete acid suppression. The occasional reflux episodes experienced by many patients on 40 mg of omeprazole per day may be "normal" and not significant; however, in patients with LPR, especially voice professionals, any laryngeal acid exposure is detrimental. Rather than doing 24-hour pH monitoring studies on medication for every patient with LPR or prescribing even higher doses of PPIs routinely, some physicians recommend antacids, H_2 blockers, and/or lifestyle modifications in addition to PPIs. The antacids are used at bedtime and before strenuous exercise (such as singing). This regimen may be useful for singers in whom the laryngeal appearance improves but incompletely with PPI therapy.

More recently, in treating patients with LPR, a PPI has been combined with an H_2 blocker at bedtime, for reasons discussed next. Clearly, research into optimal treatment regimens is needed.

H_2-RECEPTOR ANTAGONISTS

Since their introduction in the late 1970s, H_2-receptor antagonists have been the mainstay of treatment for GERD. The only mechanism of action of these drugs is to inhibit gastric acid secretion; they have no effect on LES pressure or esophageal clearance. The 4 H_2 blockers—cimetidine, ranitidine, famotidine, and nizatidine—are equal in efficacy when used in equivalent doses. These agents are extremely well tolerated in all age groups and produce complete relief of heartburn in 60% of patients treated.[13] Healing of mucosal abnormalities in the esophagus is less frequent and often overestimated, being seen in 0% to 82% (mean 48%) of patients.[13] The best results are seen in patients with nonerosive esophagitis, in whom success rates are as high as 75%.[13] Higher doses of H_2 antagonists, up to 4 times daily, are usually needed to treat erosive esophagitis[15]; however, the cost of this double-dose therapy is greater and therapy is not as clinically effective as use of a single daily dose of a PPI. Maintenance of heartburn relief and healing of esophageal mucosal injury are seen in only 25% to 50% of patients receiving continuous therapy at traditional doses of H_2 antagonists (eg, ranitidine 150 mg twice daily) for 1 year.[16]

H_2-receptor antagonists are remarkably safe agents. Side effects are rarely seen with greater frequency than noted with placebo in clinical trials. Rare cases of hepatitis, qualitative platelet defects, and mental confusion with intravenous administration have been reported. Drug interactions are extremely rare, although they seem to be slightly more prevalent with cimetidine. Caution should be exercised in patients on dilantin, warfarin, or theophylline therapy, although clinically problems are rare.[17]

Cimetidine has also been associated with male infertility. Although the cause-and-effect relationship has not been proved, impotence and gynecomastia have also been reported as possible complications. An uncontrolled study by Van Thiel et al[18] reported that the concentration of sperm in 7 men was reduced during treatment with cimetidine (Tagamet) 300 mg 4 times daily for 9 weeks. In only 1 patient did the count fall below the lower limit of normal of 50,000,000/mL (ie, to 45,000,000/mL). After the treatment period, the concentrations returned to pretreatment levels. In contrast, in a controlled double-blind study by Enzmann et al[19] of the effects of cimetidine on spermatogenesis, 30 normal men who received cimetidine (300 mg 4 times daily or 400 mg at bedtime) or placebo for 6 months demonstrated no effects on spermatogenesis, sperm count, motility, morphology, or fertilizing capacity in vitro. Blood levels of androgen and gonadotropin were unchanged.

Carlson et al[20] studied the endocrine effects of cimetidine after acute and chronic administration in both men and women. These investigators noted the rise in prolactin levels after the acute intravenous administration of cimetidine (Tagamet). However, no acute change in the prolactin levels was noted after oral administration (300 mg cimetidine) or intravenous injection (50 mg cimetidine). The patients taking cimetidine on a chronic oral basis experienced no significant changes in serum prolactin, testosterone, free testosterone, estradiol, luteinizing hormone, or follicle-stimulating hormone. The authors concluded that it is likely that the impotence and breast changes occasionally seen during cimetidine therapy are due to peripheral antagonism of androgen action rather than to alterations in circulating hormone levels.

Winters et al[21] analyzed the effects of cimetidine on androgen binding in human prostate, testes, and semen. They found that cimetidine competed for dihydrotestosterone-binding sites in the human prostate, with no apparent binding in the testes or semen. In agreement with Carlson et al, these authors postulate that androgen antagonism may be the mechanism of the endocrine side effects of cimetidine in humans.

Jensen and coworkers[22] studied the use of cimetidine to determine the long-term effectiveness of medical management in 22 patients with gastric hypersecretory states (20 patients had Zollinger-Ellison syndrome, and 2 had idiopathic hypersecretion). Of the 22 patients followed, 11 reported impotence, breast tenderness, or gynecomastia, or some combination of these. The remaining 11 patients were asymptomatic. The mean dose of cimetidine in the patients with impotence or breast changes tended to be higher than that in patients without these side effects (5.3 ± 3.5 vs 3.0 ± 1.3 g per day). This dosage is more than 4 times that used in the therapy of uncomplicated gastric or duodenal ulcers, where impotence and gynecomastia have been reported extremely rarely.

Malagelada et al[23] also studied the long-term use of cimetidine in 18 patients with Zollinger-Ellison syndrome. The patients received an average cimetidine dosage of 2.0 g per day for an average of 28.9 months (range, 7–59 mo). In contrast to Jensen's findings, none of these patients presented with major side effects. There were no reports of impotence among this group; however, 1 patient developed tender gynecomastia.

These problems have not been reported prominently with other H_2 antagonists (which have not been studied as extensively), but complications can occur with all the medications in this class, and physicians should be familiar with them. It is also helpful to warn patients that H_2-receptor antagonists may result in increased blood alcohol levels and functional impairment after consumption of amounts of alcohol that would be considered safe in the absence of H_2-receptor antagonist therapy. This problem is particularly prominent with cimetidine.[24]

There are few trials in which H_2-receptor antagonists have been evaluated systematically in the treatment of extraesophageal GERD, and all the reported trials have been in patients with either asthma or chronic cough. The largest study, by Larrain et al,[25] randomized patients to placebo, cimetidine 300 mg 4 times a day, or antireflux surgery in a 6-month treatment trial. Most of the patients had mild GERD; before treatment, heartburn was reported less than once a week by all patients, and 66% had no evidence of esophagitis on endoscopic examination. All patients had abnormal esophageal acid exposure during prolonged pH monitoring. Both pulmonary and esophageal symptoms were decreased in the cimetidine and surgery groups compared with the placebo group. However, the response to surgical therapy was statistically superior to that obtained with medical therapy. Response to cimetidine was slower in patients with extraesophageal reflux than in typical patients with heartburn, with many patients achieving optimal response only after 4 to 6 months of treatment.[25]

Another study, comparing ranitidine 150 mg 3 times daily with antireflux surgery, showed a statistical advantage for antireflux surgery.[26] These studies reinforce the view that the superior control of esophageal acid exposure seen after antireflux surgery, compared with the control by H_2 blockers, may be needed for optimal relief of pulmonary (and other extraesophageal) symptoms. Several other short-term studies using H_2-receptor antagonists in doses ranging from 150 mg of ranitidine at bedtime to 150 mg 3 times a day for periods of 1 to 8 weeks have consistently demonstrated relief of heartburn. However, they demonstrate limited improvement in objective changes of pulmonary function and limited decrease in symptoms at the end of these 8-week trials.[27–29] Decreases in respiratory symptoms, if they occurred, lagged weeks behind decreases in esophageal symptoms. Clinical experience confirms these findings.

Cimetidine has been used successfully in unblinded and uncontrolled trials in patients with chronic cough associated with GERD. Decreased coughing has been reported in 70% to 100%.[30–33] Time to symptom reduction was quite prolonged, usually about 161 to 179 days. Patients with heartburn as the primary GERD symptom usually improve in 1 to 3 weeks. Despite reports of clinical improvement, no correlation was seen between clinical response and reduction in esophageal acid exposure by prolonged pH monitoring, which was performed at the end of the study. Although H_2 blockers were used extensively before the introduction of PPIs, there are no definitive studies in which H_2 blockers have been used to treat LPR. Currently we use them in patients who are unable to tolerate PPIs and in those who have symptoms from nocturnal acid secretion despite the use of PPIs. If H_2 blockers are to be used, high-dose therapy is required, using as a minimum the equivalent dose of ranitidine 150 mg 4 times a day (Table 8–2). We also use H_2 blockers (ranitidine 300 mg) at bedtime to control nocturnal acid breakthrough that may occur even in patients taking high doses of PPIs.

PROKINETIC AGENTS

Drugs that increase LES pressure and accelerate esophageal clearance and gastric emptying are ideal agents to "correct" the pathogenic problems underlying GERD. Unfortunately, the results seen with the 2 most commonly prescribed prokinetic agents, metoclopramide and cisapride, have been somewhat disappointing in treating GERD. Equal efficacy is seen with these agents. Heartburn relief can be achieved with cisapride in close to 60% of patients when 10 mg is given 4 times a day and is equal in efficacy to H_2-receptor antagonists.[34] Studies suggest that comparable heartburn relief can be achieved with 20 mg twice a day, a dosage that will increase compliance.[35]

Metoclopramide is the only available motility agent in the United States, in a new tablet (including oral disintegrating) and liquid form. The drug has been reported to sensitize tissues to the action of acetyl-

Table 8–2. Standard Medical Therapy of Gastroesophageal Reflux

Agents	Dosage
Prokinetic (promotility) agents	
Metoclopramide	5–10 mg 4 times a day
Cisapride	10 mg 4 times a day
Acid suppressive agents	
H2-receptor antagonists*	
Cimetidine	400 mg 2 times a day (nonerosive symptomatic disease) 800 mg 2 times a day (erosive esophagitis)
Ranitidine	150 mg 2 times a day (nonerosive symptomatic disease) 150 mg 4 times a day (erosive esophagitis)
Famotidine	20 mg 2 times a day (nonerosive symptomatic disease) 40 mg 2 times a day (erosive esophagitis)
Nizatidine	150 mg 2 times a day (all forms of reflux disease)
Proton-pump inhibitors†	
Omeprazole	20 mg a day acute and maintenance therapy
Lansoprazole	30 mg a day (acute) 15 mg a day (maintenance)
Pantoprazole	40 mg a day (acute and maintenance)
Esomeprazole	20–40 mg once daily (healing phase) 20 mg a day (maintenance)
Rabeprazole	20 mg a day (acute and maintenance)

*Also available over the counter in reduced dose for medication as needed.

†Higher doses are required for treatment of extraesophageal disease. See text.

choline and has been shown in some studies to increase the amplitude of gastric and esophageal contractions, increase LES pressure, and accelerate gastric emptying. Equivalent in efficacy to H_2-receptor antagonists and superior to placebo at a dosage of 10 mg 4 times daily for heartburn and other GERD symptoms, no effective healing of erosive esophagitis can be shown superior to placebo. Clinically important central nervous system side effects, such as drowsiness and confusion, and serious side effects like anxiety, agitation, confusion, motor restlessness, hallucinations, depression, and tardive dyskinesia (potentially irreversible) make it a difficult drug to use in any GERD patient. Side effects are likely dose related and may be worse in children and the elderly. This agent has a black box warning for side effects, and informed written consent is to be considered if prescribed for long-term use. When gastroparesis and GERD symptoms refractory to antisecretory therapy coexist, metoclopramide may be of additional benefit. There is little evidence to support empiric use of this agent as an add-on to PPIs in the absence of delayed gastric emptying. Our preference is to start with a low dose (5 mg 2–4 times a day) and titrate up for GERD. There is little need to consider this drug for the LPR patient.

Prokinetic agents have been used alone or in combination therapy with H2 antagonists for treatment of cough, predominantly in children, but they have not been extensively studied in the treatment of cough-related asthma and/or LPR. Decreased coughing was seen in 64.5% to 100% of patients in 2 uncontrolled studies.[37,38] These studies used cisapride, which is no longer available for use in the United States. The data are presented for completeness. Cisapride was studied in 22 infants aged 4 to 26 weeks with abnormal sleep pattern characterized by apneic episodes and associated GERD by pH monitoring,[39] as well as a group of 19 children aged 3 months to 10 years (mean, 7 y) with either nocturnal cough, wheezing, or bronchitis, all of whom also had GERD confirmed by pH monitoring.[40] Apnea, night cough, and asthma symptoms were decreased in 70% to 90%. Objectively, GERD was decreased as confirmed by pH monitoring after treatment. A third study evaluating the use of cisapride in 27 children (mean age, 6 y) with refractory asthma and GERD confirmed by pH monitoring reported partial or complete relief of respiratory symptoms in 80% after 3 months of treatment.[41]

A recent preliminary study by Khoury et al,[42] a double-blind controlled trial in 16 adult patients with pulmonary symptoms and GERD documented by ambulatory pH monitoring, compared cisapride 10 mg 4 times a day with placebo. Significant improvement in forced expiratory volume in 1 second and forced vital capacity was noted in patients on cisapride compared with placebo. No improvement in objective assessment of esophageal acid exposure by ambulatory pH monitoring or in esophageal symptoms could be documented. Prokinetic agents have not been studied for efficacy in patients with LPR.

PROTON-PUMP INHIBITORS

As Altman and Radosevich[43] pointed out, although H_2 receptor blockers are still used, PPI therapy is the most effective and most widely used nonsurgical treatment for GERD and LPR. PPIs—omeprazole, lansoprazole, rabeprazole, pantoprazole, dexlansoprazole, and esomeprazole—inhibit the H+/K+ATPase enzyme that catalyzes the terminal step of acid secretion in the parietal cells. Profound acid inhibition is possible with these agents, resulting in improved symptom relief and healing of erosive disease. A single daily dose of either omeprazole or rabeprazole produces a 67% to 95% (mean 83%) rate of symptom relief and healing of erosive esophagitis.[44,45] A large trial comparing omeprazole 20 mg daily with lansoprazole 30 mg daily showed comparable healing rates of over 85% after 8 weeks of therapy.[46] Successful, complete symptom relief and healing of erosive esophagitis are seen in 85% of patients when continuous therapy is given over 1 year.[47] Continuous therapy with omeprazole is significantly superior to alternate-day or weekend therapy and to H_2-receptor antagonist therapy in the long-term treatment of GERD. Continuous therapy with omeprazole 20 to 60 mg a day has been shown to maintain complete symptom relief and healing for up to 5 years, even in patients refractory to H_2 antagonists.[48] This study illustrates several key points: long-term remission is possible in up to 100% of patients if adequate doses of PPIs are used; up to 30% of patients with GERD refractory to H_2 antagonists require either twice-daily or more frequent dosing of PPIs; and most patients respond to stable doses of omeprazole given as long-term therapy without the development of tolerance. A preliminary report of continued follow-up of this same patient group shows continued success of omeprazole for 11 years. Relapse occurred in 1 patient after 9 years of treatment, with minimal side effects.[49]

Combination therapy with PPIs and prokinetics is used commonly in patients whose reflux is difficult to manage. Unfortunately, no studies have shown a statistical advantage for combination therapy over increasing the dose of PPIs, which appear to have their best effect when given a half hour to an hour before a meal—and if more than a single dose is required, they should be given in divided doses twice daily before breakfast and dinner[50,51] or more frequently. Omission of breakfast will reduce the efficacy of PPIs.[52] If PPIs are used in combination with antacids, the medications should be separated by about an hour, with the antacids being taken about a half-hour after meals. If an H_2 antagonist is added, it should be given at bedtime. Recent data suggest that combining a PPI twice daily with an H_2 antagonist at bedtime may be particularly helpful. Peghini et al[53] demonstrated nocturnal gastric acid breakthrough between 2 AM and 5 AM in a majority of patients and normal volunteers taking a PPI twice daily. In a follow-up study, Peghini et al[54] suggested that this nocturnal acid breakthrough is histamine related, and they demonstrated that an H_2 blocker (ranitidine 300 mg) at bedtime is more effective than bedtime omeprazole for controlling residual nocturnal acid secretion.

In certain clinical situations, difficulty in swallowing mandates an alternative method of administering PPIs. Multiple studies with omeprazole and 2 studies with lansoprazole have shown that these PPIs can be given to patients who are unable to ingest intact capsules by opening the capsule and mixing the intact granules with water, which results in a bicarbonate-based suspension. They can also be put in apple or orange juice, or the granules can be sprinkled on applesauce or yogurt. The capsules should not be crushed.[55] Adequate control of intragastric pH has been demonstrated when omeprazole suspension is given via percutaneous gastrostomy, jejunostomy, or nasogastric tube. This mode of administration is particularly useful in postoperative patients prone to aspiration, patients at risk for stress ulceration, and patients receiving chronic enteral feeding via gastrostomy tube.

Since omeprazole and lansoprazole were introduced, additional PPIs have become available. Rabeprazole, pantoprazole, dexlansoprazole, and esomeprazole have slightly different pharmacokinetic profiles, and they have been studied less extensively than omeprazole and lansoprazole; but all 5 PPIs appear effective for treatment of GERD and probably LPR as well. Omeprazole has been studied for treatment of posterior laryngitis and was found to decrease symptoms and signs of LPR.[56] It is important to recognize that symptoms abate before signs in most cases. A recent study by Belafsky et al[57] supports this common clinical observation. They noted that symptoms resolved maximally during the first 2 months of therapy, but laryngeal appearance improved slightly during the first 2 months and continued improving for at least the first 6 months of therapy.

PPIs have an excellent safety profile, with no side effects other than those seen with placebo as reported in clinical trials. The major side effects, headache and diarrhea, are quite rare. There has been concern about long-term safety of PPIs because of their profound acid suppression. Current evidence suggests that this fear is unjustified, as ample gastric acid is produced in a 24-hour period to allow for normal protein digestion and for iron and calcium absorption, to prevent bacterial overgrowth, and to maintain vitamin B_{12} absorption. The most important concerns with long-term use of PPIs are hyperplasia of enterochromaffin-like cells and development of gastric carcinoid tumors resulting from hypersecretion of gastrin. There have been no reports of gastric carcinoid or any gastric malignancy with up to 11 years of omeprazole therapy.[49] Hyperplasia of enterochromaffin-like cells is seen in 4% or fewer of patients receiving PPIs. A recent study suggested that in patients on long-term omeprazole therapy who were infected with *Helicobacter pylori*, atrophic gastritis (a proposed precursor of gastric adenocarcinoma) developed at a more rapid rate than in patients who were not infected, prompting the authors to recommend screening for and treatment of *H. pylori* infection in patients on long-term therapy with PPIs.[58] A Food and Drug Administration (FDA) panel determined that these data are insufficient to support this recommendation.[59] No specific laboratory monitoring—in particular, of serum gastrin—is required for patients on long-term PPIs.

Side Effects

Potential side effects associated with PPI therapy include headache, diarrhea, and dyspepsia in <2% of users. Switching to another PPI can be considered if this occurs. More recently, new discussions have been raised regarding associations with vitamin and mineral deficiencies, new data on infections, including community-acquired pneumonia and *Clostridium difficile*, infection and the extensive literature on associations of PPI use, with long bone fractures, and cardiovascular events in patients receiving concomitant therapy with clopidogrel (Plavix). Clopidogrel is a platelet activation inhibitor used as a "blood thinner" in many patients with cardiovascular disorders, often in association with aspirin (see the section "Suggested approach to treatment of laryngopharyngeal reflux" later in this chapter). The FDA issued warnings regarding the potential for adverse cardiovascular events among clopidogrel users taking PPI therapy in 2009 and regarding the potential for wrist, hip, and spine fractures among PPI users in 2010. In late 2012, the FDA issued a class warning for *C. difficile* infections.

Two recent reviews demonstrated evidence that PPI therapy reduces the absorption of protein-bound vitamin B_{12}, but not enough clinical evidence to document B_{12} deficiency in chronic PPI users or the need to check B_{12} levels. Recent studies have suggested that in elderly institutionalized long-term PPI users, B_{12} deficiency is more likely to develop and should be considered.[60,61]

Gastric acid is needed to allow absorption of non-heme iron and enhance iron salt dissociation from ingested food. Iron deficiency anemia has been reported in patients with atrophic gastritis, gastric resection, or vagotomy. To date, no data are available demonstrating the development of iron deficiency anemia in normal subjects on PPI therapy.

By their effects in increasing gastric pH levels, PPIs may encourage growth of gut microflora and increase susceptibility to organisms such as *Salmonella*, *Campylobacter jejuni*, *Escherichia coli*, *C. difficile*, *Vibrio cholerae*, and *Listeria*. An increased susceptibility in PPI users for *Salmonella*, *Campylobacter*, and *C. difficile* infections was found in a systematic review.[60,62] Current recommendations are to carefully evaluate the need for PPI therapy in hospitalized patients who need intravenous antibiotics to reduce risk for *C. difficile*.

An increased risk for community-acquired pneumonia is difficult to demonstrate in association with PPI therapy. A meta-analysis showed that the overall risk for pneumonia was higher among users of PPIs. If only randomized controlled trial data are analyzed, H_2-receptor antagonists rather than PPIs have been associated with an elevated risk for hospital-acquired pneumonia.[63] A more recent meta-analysis did find an increased risk for pneumonia associated with PPI use, but the results were confounded by methodologic issues. Paradoxically, short duration of use was associated with increased odds of community-acquired pneumonia but chronic use was not.[64] No definite recommendation can be given in this complex area.

Clinical studies in patients taking PPI therapy have shown mixed results regarding fracture. The study with the longest clinical follow-up matched cases with abnormal bone mineral density (osteoporosis) at the hip or lumbar vertebrae (T-score ≤ -2.5) to controls with normal bone mineral density (T-score ≥ 1.0). PPI use was not associated with having osteoporosis in either the hip or the lumbar spine for PPI use >1500 doses over the previous 5 years. In the longitudinal study, no significant decrease was observed in bone mineral density at either site attributable to PPI use. This suggests that the association between PPI use and hip fracture was probably related to factors independent of osteoporosis.[65]

In a recent meta-analysis, the pooled odds ratio (OR) for fracture was 1.29 (95% confidence interval [CI], 1.18–1.41) with PPIs and 1.10 (95% CI, 0.99–1.23) with H_2-receptor antagonist use compared with nonuse. Another study showed that the hip fracture risk among PPI users was seen only in persons with at least one other fracture-risk factor.[66] A meta-analysis covering 1,521,062 patients showed significant risk for spine fractures (OR, 1.50; 95% CI, 1.32–1.72; p <.001). For hip fractures, there was an increased risk for fractures with PPIs (OR, 1.23; 95% CI, 1.11–1.36; p <.001). Overall, an OR of 1.20 is seen for PPIs, and an OR of 1.08 is seen for H_2-receptor antagonists (95% CI, 1.00–1.18; p +0.06).

Again, short duration of PPI use may be associated with increased risk for developing hip fracture (OR, 1.24; 95% CI, 1.19–1.28), but not in long-term PPI users (OR, 1.30; 95% CI, 0.98–1.70).[67] No change in bone mineral density was seen in patients using PPIs continuously for 5 to 10 years in a Canadian study[68] despite the finding of a lower baseline bone mineral density in those same patients.

In 2009, the FDA issued a warning regarding the potential for increased adverse cardiovascular events in concomitant users of PPIs and clopidogrel, particularly users of omeprazole, lansoprazole, and esomeprazole. In vitro, the antiplatelet activity of clopidogrel requires activation by cytochrome (CY)P2C19, which is the same pathway through which PPIs are metabolized. Although overall studies have been conflicting, the newest data suggest that dexlansoprazole does not inhibit platelets in vitro to the same degree as do the 3 former PPIs. Pantoprazole appears to have less inhibition as well. A recent meta-analysis (27 studies) focused on primary myocardial infarction, stroke, stent occlusion, death, and secondary outcomes (rehospitalization for cardiac symptoms or revascularization procedures).[68] Outcomes from the 2 randomized controlled trials did not show an increased risk for adverse outcomes. Meta-analysis of primary and secondary outcomes showed an increased risk difference for all studies. Essentially, the risk for adverse cardiac outcomes was 0% based on data from well-controlled randomized trials.[70] Data from retrospective studies and the addition of probable vascular events slightly but significantly increased the risk estimates, likely due to lack of adjustment for potential confounders. Recent consensus is that PPIs can be used with clopidogrel if they are clinically indicated.

Several clinical trials have been conducted using PPIs in patients with extraesophageal symptoms, principally asthma and LPR. All the early trials were conducted with omeprazole. Two short-term studies—one with omeprazole 20 mg once a day for 4 weeks[71] and the other with omeprazole 20 mg twice daily for 6 weeks[72]—showed an improvement in pulmonary function parameters with omeprazole therapy compared with placebo. However, little change in bronchodilator use or asthma scores could be demonstrated. A longer, randomized double-blind controlled trial in 36 patients by Boeree et al[73] comparing omeprazole 40 mg twice daily with placebo for 3 months showed a reduction in nocturnal cough during treatment with omeprazole compared with placebo. However, objective changes in forced expiratory volume in 1 second and other indices of pulmonary function were not seen.[74]

The study by Meier et al[72] using omeprazole 20 mg twice daily found that 6 of 11 patients who failed to improve on omeprazole also did not experience healing of their esophagitis. This finding suggests that acid suppression was inadequate in these patients. The patients in whom control of asthma was obtained also demonstrated healing of their esophagitis, reinforcing the principle that adequate acid control can relieve pulmonary symptoms.

Important insights into the treatment of patients with extraesophageal GERD come from a well-designed study by Harding et al[75] in which 30 patients with documented asthma and proven GERD by prolonged pH monitoring received increasing doses of omeprazole beginning with 20 mg a day, increasing by 20 mg daily after every 8 weeks of treatment for 3 months, or until esophageal acid exposure was reduced to "normal." Normalization of esophageal acid exposure resulted in reduction in pulmonary symptoms in 70% of patients. There are several important observations from this trial: 8 of 30 patients (28%) required more than 20 mg of omeprazole daily to normalize esophageal acid exposure; many patients required the entire 3-month period of treatment to achieve optimal symptom relief, with improvement progressing continuously over the 3-month period; a favorable response to omeprazole was seen in patients who presented with frequent regurgitation (more than once a week) or abnormal proximal acid exposure demonstrated by ambulatory pH monitoring, or both (see Chapter 6). The study emphasizes the importance of adequate esophageal acid control to achieve improvement in patients with extraesophageal symptoms. Complete elimination of esophageal acid exposure is often necessary in patients with extraesophageal disease (including LPR) to effectively relieve symptoms. The authors require that esophageal pH be >4 for 99% of the time of prolonged pH monitoring during PPI therapy before accepting that acid suppression is optimal. In selected cases, even this criterion is not adequate in patients with LPR if the 1% period of reflux includes proximal acid exposure with persistent laryngeal symptoms and signs.

Kamel et al[56] evaluated 16 patients with posterior laryngitis (ie, LPR) who had failed to respond to initial treatment with conservative lifestyle measures for a 6-week period on omeprazole 40 mg daily for at least 6 weeks. Laryngeal and esophageal symptom scores improved significantly at the end of 6 weeks compared with preomeprazole scores. Objective improvement over pretreatment values was also seen when the larynx was evaluated by a blinded investigator using videolaryngoscopy. Six patients had improvement in their laryngoscopic scores but not laryngeal symptom scores. Symptoms recurred within 6 weeks in all patients after therapy was stopped. Poorer response was seen in patients with abnormal proximal esophageal acid exposure on ambulatory pH monitoring. It is reasonable to speculate that 40 mg a day of omeprazole was inadequate therapy for these patients and that they might have responded to higher doses or to a regimen combining other medications.

The same investigators studied 182 patients with posterior laryngitis and at least one of the following symptoms: postnasal drip, persistent or recurrent sore throat, cough, or hoarseness.[76] Patients were treated sequentially with conservative lifestyle modifications for an initial period of 6 to 12 weeks, followed by famotidine 20 mg at bedtime for an additional 6 weeks. Omeprazole 20 mg at bedtime was given to nonresponders. Omeprazole was then increased in 20-mg increments every 6 weeks until a dose of 80 mg a day was reached. Laryngitis was characterized as mild if posterior laryngeal erythema was seen; moderate if marked erythema, secretions, and mucosal granularity were present; or severe if ulceration, granulation tissue, or hyperkeratosis was seen. Patients with mild symptoms and minimal laryngeal changes responded to conservative doses of famotidine, whereas patients with severe laryngitis required PPIs.[76]

These studies underscore variability in response of patients with LPR, the need to treat for longer periods before seeing a response when disease is severe, the need for higher doses of PPIs, and the rapid recurrence of symptoms when therapy is discontinued, emphasizing that long-term treatment is often needed in patients with LPR.

Wo et al[77] studied 22 patients with posterior laryngitis thought to be secondary to GERD and diagnosed by indirect laryngoscopy, using an 8-week trial of omeprazole 40 mg at bedtime. Laryngeal symptoms decreased in 67% of these patients. Increasing the omeprazole dosage to 40 mg twice a day in nonresponders did not improve the response. Relapse was seen in 40% when omeprazole was stopped. There were no predictors of response, although nocturnal symptoms were more common in nonresponders. Perhaps this group had nocturnal acid breakthrough and continued to experience reflux despite high-dose PPI therapy. It is likely that results would have been improved if omeprazole had been given twice daily (before breakfast and dinner), a treatment regimen that produces acid suppression superior to that obtained with other modes of administration of this drug.[77] The response rate to omeprazole in this trial does, however, support empiric therapy for LPR.

Metz and colleagues[78] studied 10 patients with laryngitis documented by endoscopy who also had GERD diagnosed by ambulatory pH monitoring. They used 40 mg omeprazole as a single daily dose and found improvement in 7 of 10 patients (70%) at the end of 8 weeks. Jaspersen and colleagues[79]studied 34 patients with laryngeal symptoms, laryngoscopic changes of LPR, and erosive esophagitis who received omeprazole 20 mg a day for 4 weeks, and the authors reported healing of esophagitis and reduction in laryngeal symptoms in 32 of the 34 patients (92%). No comment was made about laryngeal examinations. The latter 3 studies[77,78,79] were uncontrolled but showed excellent results with omeprazole. Although lansoprazole has not been studied in this patient population, comparable healing rates for omeprazole 20 mg a day and lansoprazole 30 mg a day are seen in erosive esophagitis,[46] suggesting that this PPI should be as effective as omeprazole in patients with LPR and other extraesophageal disease.

El-Serag and Sonnenberg[80] performed a randomized controlled trial in 20 patients with LPR comparing lansoprazole 30 mg twice daily with placebo. After 16 weeks, 50% of the treated patients had complete relief of LPR symptoms, compared with 10% with placebo. Laryngeal findings were not highlighted.

A prospective, placebo-controlled study of PPI therapy for patients with LPR was published by El-Serag et al[81] in which 22 patients from a Veteran's Administration hospital population were treated with lansoprazole 30 mg twice daily or placebo for 3 months. Subjects underwent esophagoscopy, 24-hour pH monitor studies, and indirect laryngoscopy using a laryngeal telescope. The lower sensor was 5 cm above the LES, and the sensors were separated by 15 cm. Their primary outcome criterion was complete resolution of laryngeal symptoms. Of the 20 patients (out of 22) who finished the study and had all information available, 11 received lansoprazole and 9 received placebo. Seven patients were complete responders, 6 of whom received lansoprazole and 1 of whom received placebo. The difference was statistically significant. At the end of this study, 58% of the patients treated with lansoprazole had complete (n = 2) or partial (n = 5) resolution of laryngeal signs of reflux (posterior laryngitis), and 30% of the placebo-treated group had partial resolution of laryngeal signs (none had complete resolution). The authors concluded that lansoprazole is effective in the treatment of LPR. The study was well designed, but the population was fairly small; and a VA hospital population is not necessarily comparable with the general population (21/22 subjects were male; mean age was 59 y in the lansoprazole group and 65 y in the placebo group).

In 2001, Noordzij et al[82] reported on 53 patients with reflux laryngitis. Of these, 30 subjects were enrolled, who had more than 4 episodes of proximal reflux during their 24-hour monitor study. Fifteen received omeprazole 40 mg twice daily, and the other 15 received placebo. The study lasted for 2 months. They assessed symptoms and laryngeal signs of LPR. During 24-hour pH monitor studies, the upper sensor was placed under flexible fiberoptic guidance 1 cm above the UES, and the distal sensor was 18 cm from the proximal sensor. The patients were instructed to avoid behavioral changes known to have an effect on gastroesophageal reflux. The mean age (y) in the treatment group was 51.7; in the placebo group, 45.3. Subjects were fairly evenly divided by gender. There were large differences in initial symptom severity between the omeprazole and placebo groups for some symptoms. The authors reported that most symptom scores improved for both groups, although mild hoarseness and throat clearing improved significantly more in the treatment group than in subjects receiving placebo. Endoscopic laryngeal signs did not change significantly in either group. They concluded that mild hoarseness and throat clearing may be treated effectively by omeprazole, but they also concluded that there was a placebo effect. It is interesting that laryngoscopic findings showed no improvement in either group. Although complete resolution of laryngeal signs commonly takes many months, improvement in erythema is usually seen in <2 months, and improvements in edema often are seen during this time as well. Their results may have been due to the fact that abnormalities in laryngeal signs were very mild in the entire study population (in blind subjective assessments, the 5 laryngeal signs were all rated in the 0–1 range). Hence, very little change in laryngeal findings could be expected. Findings might well be different in a population with more severe disease.

In 2003, Eherer et al[83] reported a placebo-controlled, double-blind crossover study of the effects of pantoprazole on LPR. They assessed 62 patients. Twenty-four showed reflux on 24-hour pH monitoring, and 21 were entered into the study. The proximal sensor was located 1 to 3 cm above the UES, and the distal sensor was placed 15, 18, or 21 cm below the upper sensor. Studies monitoring pH were performed for each subject prior to entry into the study and between its two 3-month arms. The requirement for 2 pH monitoring studies, and the duration of the study (>6 months) may be responsible for the fact that only 14 patients completed all portions of the research protocol. All subjects were nonsmokers. However, the methodology makes no mention of preventing patients from adopting behavioral changes that might have contributed to improvements in both groups. The authors reported that both pantoprazole and placebo were associated with "marked improvement" in laryngitis scores and that there was no significant difference between the 2 treatments after 3 months. After a 2-week washout period, a second pH monitoring study confirmed persistence of reflux in most subjects. Switching the placebo group to pantoprazole resulted in further improvement of laryngitis scores. In the pantoprazole group switched to placebo, a minority of patients had recurrence of symptoms and signs. Changes in symptom scores were not significantly different between the 2 treatment groups. After reversal of treatments, there was also no significant change in symptoms, although 1 patient who switched from pantoprazole to placebo had a severe recurrence of symptoms. Like the Noordzij et al[82] study, these results are somewhat difficult to interpret because of the fairly mild severity of LPR in both groups. For example, the maximum possible score for esophageal symptoms was 48 (the higher, the worse). The esophageal score prior to treatment in the placebo/pantoprazole group was 11.0, and in the pantoprazole/placebo group 3.3.

Similarly, the maximum laryngeal symptom score was 72. The pretreatment placebo/pantoprazole score was 17.4, and the pantoprazole/placebo score was 14.6. Hence, there was not much room for improvement; and these patients had mild disease, in which spontaneous fluctuations in severity are common. This problem, combined with the small number of subjects, raises questions about the conclusions of this otherwise well-designed study from which the authors deduced that pantoprazole may be helpful in relieving acute symptoms but that the advantage of long-term treatment has been overestimated. Substantially larger numbers and inclusion of patients with long-term, moderate-to-severe symptoms and signs will be needed to assess these concerns definitively.

Other recent studies on LPR also have failed to provide incontestable answers to questions about diagnostic accuracy and treatment efficiency.[84,85]

Bruley des Varannes et al[86] reported that the superiority of PPIs over other drugs has been well established for both short- and long-term treatment of GERD. Patients with erosive esophagitis are more responsive to PPIs than patients with nonerosive reflux disease. PPIs also have become widely used and have been proven to be safe and effective in the management of GERD in children, although to date, only omeprazole, lansoprazole, and esomeprazole are approved for use in children.[87,88]

A randomized placebo-controlled study revealed improved LPR symptoms compared with placebo after 12 weeks of treatment with rabeprazole 20 mg twice daily.[89] The authors reported a relapse of symptoms 6 weeks after stopping PPI therapy, suggesting that LPR requires longer duration of treatment. Many clinicians still advocate the use of empiric therapy with twice-daily PPI dosing for 6 to 12 weeks (on average) as a diagnostic tool in patients with suspected LPR.[90,91] However, we believe that this is not an adequate approach, particularly for nonresponders, as some patients may produce acid even when taking 2 or more PPIs daily. Monitoring of pH while on medications is invaluable in detecting these patients; and for many patients, PPI treatment must be continued indefinitely.

Dadabhai and Friedenberg[92] reported that rabeprazole has a faster onset of action in comparison with other PPIs. They cited rabeprazole's high pKa of 5.0, which facilitates activation at a higher pH, as a possible reason for its faster onset. They described rabeprazole's pathway of metabolism as nonenzymatic, thus making it less affected by the genetic polymorphisms of the CYP2C19 on which the other PPIs depend.

In 2010, Fass et al[93] reported the results of a randomized, placebo-controlled study that evaluated the effectiveness of esomeprazole twice daily in their patients with LPR, all of whom had undergone endoscopy and pH monitor testing. Following the 3-month trial, the results revealed no significant differences in videostroboscopic reflux finding score and no significant difference in acoustic measures after treatment, comparing the esomeprazole group and the placebo group. The patients completed a voice use and quality diary and a symptom diary pretreatment and at the end of the study, and no significant differences were found in these between the 2 groups.

Clinicians must be cognizant of the fact that PPI therapy is not universally effective. Caution must be exercised in interpretation of available literature. An insightful analysis by Johnston et al[94] revealed that in a recent meta-analysis, all but 2 studies fell within a funnel plot. The only 2 that did not show PPI effect were flawed by publication bias. Meta-analyses commonly magnify inherent flaws in the included studies, and more rigorous studies need to be performed. A randomized, double-blind, placebo-controlled study[95] revealed improvement in reflux finding score and reflux symptom index after treatment with esomeprazole in both placebo and PPI groups for 6 weeks. However, diffuse laryngeal edema showed significantly greater improvement in the PPI group, and ventricular obliteration and laryngeal erythema trended toward greater improvement in the PPI group. Posterior laryngeal hypertrophy improved significantly in the PPI group only. Lifestyle modifications were not instituted, so improvement was from medical intervention. Whereas a placebo effect has been shown repeatedly, including in this study, improvements were greater in the PPI group in several parameters.

Failure rates are high in patients receiving a PPI only once daily.[96,97] In addition, a morning dose of omeprazole has been shown to last an average of only 13.8 hours.[98] The problem of nocturnal acid breakthrough, discussed previously, may be viewed as effectively limiting the duration of effect for the evening dose of PPI to a period of 7½ hours.[53] In addition, a few patients demonstrate substantial (or normal) acid levels even when receiving high doses of PPIs.[97,99] Amin et al[96] studied LPR patients receiving PPIs up to 4 times a day and reported a medical treatment failure rate of 10%.

Belafsky et al[100] describe the presence of esophagopharyngeal reflux—as distinct from LPR—which should also be considered as a possible cause for treatment failures. This disorder is characterized by regurgitation of proximal esophageal contents into the laryngopharynx secondary to inadequate volume clearance and dysmotility, rather than acid and peptic injury. Further studies are needed to elucidate this process, as treatment with antireflux medications, prokinetics, dilatation, and diet modification ameliorates symptoms in 50% of affected individuals.[100]

HELICOBACTER PYLORI

If a decision is made to treat for *H. pylori* infection after the presence of this organism has been proven, a combination of agents is used. Triple therapy with clarithromycin, metronidazole, and a PPI has been reported to be efficacious, and there are few side effects.[101] Youssef et al[102] reported that 57% of their 212 patients diagnosed with LPR tested positive for the *H. pylori* stool antigen (HPSA). HPSA-negative patients were treated with esomeprazole alone, and 96.6% improved. HPSA-positive patients were divided into 2 groups. Only 40% of those treated with esomeprazole alone improved, while 90% of those who received triple therapy (esomeprazole, amoxicillin, and clarithromycin) showed improvement. These findings suggest that screening and treatment for HPSA may be advisable in LPR patients, although attention to *H. pylori* is not routine in most centers. At present, our therapy consists of a PPI twice daily, clarithromycin 500 mg twice daily, and amoxicillin 1 g twice daily for 1 week.

SUGGESTED APPROACH TO TREATMENT OF LARYNGOPHARYNGEAL REFLUX

Current practice suggests that PPI therapy is the treatment of choice for patients with LPR. A starting dose of a PPI twice daily, before breakfast and dinner, for 2 to 3 months is our initial minimum treatment trial regimen. Current experience suggests that 70% of patients will respond to this therapy, although many will require long treatment periods to achieve optimal results. One of us (R.T.S.) routinely used to prescribe antacids 4 times daily for the first 3 to 4 weeks of treatment. Anecdotally, long-term treatment with H_2 blockers or PPIs has worked fairly well, with most patients remaining on antacids (as well as on PPIs or H_2 blockers) at bedtime and prior to exercise, and with only a few patients needing PPIs more than twice daily. However, since the reports by Peghini,[53,54] ranitidine 300 mg is sometimes added at bedtime to the PPIs twice daily in patients with prominent symptoms and signs of LPR. Some patients also still use antacids before strenuous exercise or singing performance.

Patients who have a good initial response to this therapeutic trial should be continued at the same dose for an additional 4- to 8-week period to assess for continued improvement. If complete symptom relief and mucosal healing are not achieved at this point, the patient should be reevaluated with prolonged ambulatory pH monitoring studies while on therapy with PPIs to assess the adequacy of intragastric acid suppression and elimination of distal and proximal esophageal acid exposure. If acid suppression is incomplete, additional medical therapy is indicated before it can be assumed that the patient experienced treatment failure. If the patient has a poor response to the initial therapeutic trial, prolonged ambulatory pH monitoring while the patient continues therapy should be performed to evaluate drug efficacy. Treatment with higher PPI doses of 3 or even 4 daily (eg, esomeprazole 80 mg before breakfast and 80 mg before dinner) may be needed to control symptoms and signs of LPR. Even on such superdoses, close 24-hour pH impedance monitoring shows that some patients will continue to reflux acid.[103] If such patients remain symptomatic, they may benefit from fundoplication even when they do not meet the generally accepted criteria for surgery.[104] If initial response to treatment is good, with resolution of symptoms and signs, long-term therapy is indicated in nearly all cases. It is reasonable to try to reduce the amount of antireflux medication, adjusting the dose as indicated by recurrence of LPR symptoms and signs. However, in our experience, the majority of patients benefit from treatment at full doses continued indefinitely. In LPR patients (especially professional singers and actors), adequate management of LPR with dietary and lifestyle modifications alone, after discontinuing medication, is unusual, except occasionally in patients who lose substantial amounts of weight.

Studies from our laboratory as cited previously have shown that 70% of patients with GERD who receive twice-daily PPI therapy will continue to have gastric acid breakthrough (pH of <4) for at least 1 hour in the overnight period.[53] Reflux will occur in 30% to 50% of these patients during this breakthrough period.[105] Another study from our laboratory found that 30% of patients with extraesophageal reflux presentations (asthma, cough, LPR) continue to have abnormal acid exposure despite therapy with a twice-daily PPI.[106] These patients require more aggressive medical therapy, as even small amounts of acid exposure may be injurious to the mucosa of the larynx, oral cavity, and airways. Doubling the dose of PPI (eg, esomeprazole 40 mg twice daily) may be sufficient to control esophageal acid exposure effectively. However, some patients will have continued nocturnal gastric acid breakthrough and esophageal reflux despite high-dose PPI therapy unless an H_2-receptor antagonist is added at night. The effectiveness of the PPI omeprazole for elimination of nocturnal breakthrough is not known. However, the prolonged antisecretory effect of this agent suggests that it may be especially useful in these patients. Ambulatory pH monitoring to document the effectiveness of therapy and to assess for the presence of continued nocturnal acid exposure is indicated if symptoms are refractory to PPIs, and especially if they persist when PPIs have been combined with an H_2-receptor antagonist.

The high prevalence of esophageal motility abnormalities, principally ineffective esophageal motility (distal esophageal contraction amplitudes <30 mm Hg in >30% of wet swallows),[107,108] in patients with extraesophageal GERD suggests that adding a prokinetic agent to therapy with a PPI should be efficacious in managing these patients. Unfortunately, there are no published data comparing combination therapy (a PPI plus cisapride or metoclopramide) with either twice-daily or higher doses of a PPI alone. Although reduction in respiratory symptoms in patients with GERD has been demonstrated in a preliminary study with cisapride, no effect on esophageal clearance, no improvement in motility abnormalities, and no change in reflux frequency can be documented in these patients.[81] We do not routinely recommend adding a prokinetic agent to therapy with PPIs. We reserve prokinetic agents for patients in whom adequate acid exposure cannot be accomplished with acid-suppressive agents and for patients with documented delayed gastric emptying.

Clinical experience suggests that most patients with LPR have chronic gastroesophageal reflux and require long-term medical therapy or antireflux surgery, or both (see Chapter 9). Of note, it is common for laryngeal reflux findings and symptoms to take longer to resolve than esophageal symptoms. Also, symptoms often improve before clinical findings, which may take 6 months or longer to reverse.[110] Reichel et al[111] noted control of LPR symptoms on daily PPI after an average of 4 weeks when combined with lifestyle modifications. Resistant cases could be treated with twice-daily medication at higher doses.[112] Improvement can be seen not only in symptoms and signs but also in objective assessments, such as acoustic parameters. Jin et al[112] reported that jitter, shimmer, and harmonic-to-noise ratio improved significantly after 1 to 2 months of treatment. The dose of PPIs and other medications and the decision to perform antireflux surgery should be individualized to maintain symptom relief and mucosal healing. Current evidence suggests that long-term medical therapy is safe and that tolerance or tachyphylaxis is extremely rare.

A recent review article[113] and editorial[114] (from which the following 9 paragraphs are adapted) highlight many of the potential problems encountered in patients who receive PPI treatment for many months or years. PPIs are fairly safe, especially compared with many other prescription drugs, but adverse effects occur and should be known to physicians who prescribe PPIs. In 2008, Davies et al[115] studied almost 12,000 patients treated with esomeprazole over an 8-month period, with an average treatment duration of 26 weeks. Only 119 events were reported as possibly related to the medication. Most were nausea and/or vomiting, diarrhea, dizziness, and headache. The few serious adverse effects were hypersensitivity reactions, including 3 cases of angioedema and 2 cases of anaphylaxis that were possibly related to the medication. This study did not examine long-term effects of PPI treatment.

PPIs are designed to cause hypochlorhydria. Therefore, they may interfere with calcium absorption. Numerous studies have confirmed that PPIs impair calcium absorption, and perhaps the best known study showed an association between PPI use and hip fracture.[116] Interestingly, Yang's study[116] showed that with long-term PPI use, risk for hip fracture was greater in men than in women. It has been speculated that this was due to the fact that many women use calcium replacement after menopause, and most men do not. At present, many of us are counseling our patients on long-term PPIs to take calcium and vitamin D supplementation while more is being learned about this problem.

Calcium absorption is not the only potential nutritional problem associated with long-term PPI use. It is also possible that vitamin B_{12} and iron levels may be affected in some patients taking PPIs for long periods of time.

Diarrhea caused by *C. difficile* has been associated with virtually all antibiotics. Recently, Aseeri et al[117] suggested that the use of PPIs may increase the risk for diarrhea under some circumstances. They felt that the inhibition of gastric acidity impaired the body's defenses against ingested bacteria. However, this study was performed in hospitalized patients, and the implications for the general healthy population remain uncertain. This is a problem that has not been encountered widely in outpatient clinical practice.

Similarly, there has been a suggestion that PPIs may be associated with an increased risk for community-acquired pneumonia. However, there are shortcomings in the papers that have studied this issue, and the conclusions of some of the studies suggesting an association remain controversial.

One of the most striking adverse effects described recently is the interaction between at least some PPIs and clopidogrel. Well-executed studies have pointed out that some PPIs reduce the biological action of clopidogrel, decreasing its effect and increasing the risk for serious cardiovascular problems, including myocardial infarction.[118,119] Clearly there is a problem with concomitant use of omeprazole and clopidogrel. This is of particular concern, not only because omeprazole is readily available over the counter, but also because many insurance companies require patients to use omeprazole (because it is inexpensive) before permitting use of a later-generation PPI. Interactions between other PPIs and clopidogrel remain under study.

Other potential adverse effects may be associated with long-term PPI use, including atrophic gastritis, possibly progressing to metaplasia and adenocarcinoma[120]; hypergastrinemia (an increase in circulating gastrin hormone that has been associated with the development of carcinoid tumors of the gastric mucosa in rats[121]); and other problems.

Although definitive information on the incidence, true causal relationship, and importance (relative to the risk for untreated LPR) of many of these adverse effects remains unknown, it is important for otolaryngologists to be aware of the potential problems associated with all of the medications we prescribe frequently.

Review of these potential problems is not intended to suggest that PPI therapy is overprescribed or should not be prescribed. The consequences of untreated LPR can be substantial and potentially life threatening. However, much of the research on adverse events of PPIs is not published in the otolaryngologic literature. Therefore, otolaryngologists have to make an extra effort to remain current on new findings so that we can counsel and treat our patients optimally. Caution should be exercised particularly when using PPIs in patients with acute coronary syndromes, and cardiology consultation should be considered when PPIs are necessary in patients taking clopidogrel.

Refractory cases may be particularly challenging. Inadequate medication dosage, resistance to medication, reactivity to nonacid reflux in adequately controlled patients, and misdiagnosis are all potential factors. Medication dosages can be increased as discussed above, as can the frequency of administration, although such modifications are "off label." Promotility agents and histamine receptor antagonists can be added. Monitoring of pH during medication can be useful in determining the cause of persistent signs and symptoms in patients receiving treatment for LPR.

Reimer et al[122] described symptom-producing rebound acid hypersecretion following withdrawal of PPI therapy after 2 months. Acid-related symptoms occurred in a group of healthy volunteers after treatment was stopped, which the authors interpreted as suggesting that rebound acid hypersecretion may result in PPI dependency. Patients who choose long-term medical therapy can be reasonably expected to avoid acid-induced mucosal injury, without risk for serious complications. Although comparison studies are inconclusive, it is likely that in most patients, long-term medical therapy with PPIs and antireflux surgery are equivalent options for minimizing acid injury, and the choice can be left to the patient in consultation with the treating physician. Acid suppression does not always provide adequate control of symptoms in patients who note symptoms from suspected pH-neutral or alkaline reflux, especially singers; although this has not been demonstrated by clinical trials, such patients may be considered for surgical therapy.

REFERENCES

1. Bell NJ, Burget DL, Howden CW, Wilkinson J, Hunt RH. Appropriate acid suppression for the management of gastro-esophageal reflux disease. *Digestion.* 1992;51(suppl 1):59–67.

2. Johnson LF, DeMeester TR. Evaluation of the head of the bed, bethanechol, and antacid form tablets on gastroesophageal reflux. *Dig Dis Sci.* 1981;26:673–680.

3. Richter JE, Castell DO. Drugs, foods, and other substances in the cause and treatment of reflux esophagitis. *Med Clin North Am.* 1981;65:1223–1234.

4. Becker DJ, Sinclair J, Castell DO, Wu WC. A comparison of high and low fat meals on postprandial esophageal acid exposure. *Am J Gastroenterol.* 1989; 84:782–786.

5. Wright LE, Castell DO. The adverse effect of chocolate on lower esophageal sphincter pressure. *Am J Dig Dis.* 1975;20:703–707.

6. Dent J, Dodds WJ, Friedman RH, et al. Mechanism of gastroesophageal reflux in recumbent asymptomatic human subjects. *J Clin Invest.* 1980;65:256–267.

7. Koufman JA. Low-acid diet for recalcitrant laryngopharyngeal reflux: therapeutic benefits and their implications. *Ann Otol Rhinol Laryngol.* 2011;120:281–287.

8. Kikendall JW, Friedman AC, Oyewole MA, et al. Pill-induced esophgeal injury: case reports and review of the medical literature. *Dig Dis Sci.* 1983;28:174–182.

9. Smoak BR, Koufman JA. Effects of gum chewing on pharyngeal and esophageal pH. *Ann Otol Rhinol Laryngol.* 2001;110:1117–1119.

10. de Groen PC, Lubbe DE, Hirsch LJ, et al. Esophagitis associated with the use of alendronate. *N Engl J Med.* 1996;335:1016–1021.

11. Kjellen G, Tibbling L, Wranne B. Effect of conservative treatment of oesophageal dysfunction in bronchial asthma. *Eur J Respir Dis.* 1981;62:190–197.

12. Katz PO. Ambulatory esophageal and hypopharyngeal pH monitoring in patients with hoarseness. *Am J Gastroenterol.* 1990;85:38–40.

13. Sontag S, Robinson M, McCallum RW, et al. Ranitidine therapy for gastroesophageal reflux disease. Results of a large double blind trial. *Arch Intern Med.* 1987;147:1485–1491.

14. McGlashan JA, Johnstone LM, Sykes J. The value of a liquid alginate suspension (Gaviscon Advance) in the management of laryngopharyngeal reflux. *Eur Arch Otorhinolaryngol.* 2009;266:243–251.

15. Euler AR, Murdock RH, Wilson TH, et al. Ranitidine is effective therapy for erosive esophagitis. *Am J Gastroenterol.* 1993;88:520–524.

16. Vigneri S, Termini R, Leandro G, et al. A comparison of five maintenance therapies for reflux esophagitis. *N Engl J Med.* 1995;333:1106–1110.

17. Feldman M, Burton ME. Histamine2-receptor antagonists: standard therapy for acid-peptic diseases. *N Engl J Med.* 1990;323:1672–1680, 1749–1755.

18. Van Thiel DH, Gavaler BS, Smith WJ Jr, Paul G. Hypothalamic-pituitary-gonadal dysfunction in men using cimetidine. *N Engl J Med.* 1979;300:1012–1015.

19. Enzmann GD, Leonard JM, Paulsen CA. Effects of cimetidine on reproductive function in men. *Clin Res.* 1981:29:26A. Abstract.

20. Carlson HE, Ippoliti AF, Swerdloff RS. Endocrine effects of acute and chronic cimetidine administration. *Dig Dis Sci.* 1981;26:428–433.

21. Winters SJ, Lee J, Troen P. Competition of the histamine H2-antagonist cimetidine for androgen binding sites in man. *J Androl.* 1980;1:111–114.

22. Jensen RT, Collen MJ, Pandol SJ, et al. Cimetidine-induced impotence and breast changes with gastric hypersecretory states. *N Engl J Med.* 1983;308:883–887.

23. Malagelada JR, Edis AJ, Adson MA, et al. Medical and surgical options in the management of patients with gastrinoma. *Gastroenterology.* 1983;84:1524–1532.

24. DiPadova C, Rome R, Frezza M, et al. Effects of ranitidine on blood alcohol levels after ethanol ingestion. *JAMA.* 1992;267:83–86.

25. Larrain A, Carrasco E, Galleguillos F, et al. Medical and surgical treatment of nonallergic asthma associated with gastroesophageal reflux. *Chest.* 1991;99:1330–1355.

26. Sontag SJ, O'Connell SA, Greenlee HB, et al. Is gastroesophageal reflux a factor in some asthmatics? *Am J Gastroenterol.* 1987;82: 119–126.

27. Harper PC, Bergner A, Kaye MD. Antireflux treatment for asthma: improvement in patients with associated gastroesophageal reflux. *Arch Intern Med.* 1987;147:56–60.

28. Ekstrom T, Lindgren BR, Tibbling L. Effects of ranitidine treatment on patients with asthma and a history of gastro-oesophageal reflux: a double blind crossover study. *Thorax.* 1989;44:19–23.

29. Gustafsson PM, Kjellman N-I, Tibbling L. A trial of ranitidine in asthmatic children and adolescents with or without pathologic gastro-oesophageal reflux. *Eur Respir J.* 1992;5:201–206.

30. Irwin RS, Curley FJ, French CL. Chronic cough: the spectrum and frequency of causes, key components of the diagnostic evaluation, and outcome of specific therapy. *Am Rev Respir Dis.* 1990;141: 640–647.

31. Irwin RS, Zawacki JK, Curley FJ, et al. Chronic cough as the sole presenting manifestation of gastroesophageal reflux. *Am Rev Respir Dis.* 1989;140:1294–1300.

32. Fitzgerald JM, Allen CJ, Craven MA, Newhouse MT. Chronic cough and gastroesophageal reflux. *Can Med Assoc J*. 1989;140:520–524.

33. Waring JP, Lacayo L, Hunter J, et al. Chronic cough and hoarseness in patients with severe gastroesophageal reflux disease. Diagnosis and response to therapy. *Dig Dis Sci*. 1995;40:1093–1097.

34. Blum AL, Adami B, Bouzo MH, et al. Effect of cisapride on relapse of esophagitis. *Dig Dis Sci*. 1993;38:551–560.

35. Castell DO, Sigmund C Jr, Patterson D, et al. Cisapride 20 mg b.i.d. provides symptomatic relief of heartburn and related symptoms of chronic mild to moderate gastroesophageal reflux disease. *Am J Gastroenterol*. 1998;93:547–552.

36. Wiseman LR, Faulds D. Cisapride: an updated review of its pharmacology and therapeutic efficacy as a prokinetic agent in gastrointestinal motility disorders. *Drugs*. 1994;47:116–152.

37. Dordal MT, Baltazar MA, Roca I, et al. Nocturnal spasmodic cough in the infant: evolution after antireflux treatment. *Allerg Immunol (Paris)*. 1994;26:53–58.

38. Dupont C, Molkhou P, Petrovic N, Fraitag B. Treatment using motilium of gastroesophageal reflux associated with respiratory manifestations in children. *Ann Pediatr (Paris)*. 1989;36:148–150.

39. Ekstrom T, Tibbling L. Esophageal acid perfusion, airway function, and symptoms in asthmatic patients with marked bronchial hyperactivity. *Chest*. 1989;96:995–998.

40. Smyrnios NA, Irwin RS, Curley FJ. Chronic cough with a history of excessive sputum production. *Chest*. 1995;108:991–997.

41. Ing AJ, Ngu MC, Breslin ABX. Chronic persistent cough and gastrooesophageal reflux. *Thorax*. 1991;46:479–483.

42. Khoury RM, Paoletti V, Cohn J, et al. Cisapride improves pulmonary function tests in patients with gastroesophageal (GE) reflux and chronic respiratory symptoms. *Gastroenterology*. 1998;114:712.

43. Altman KW, Radosevich JA. Unexpected consequences of proton pump inhibitor use. *Otolaryngol HNS*. 2009;141:564–566.

44. Sandmark S, Carlsson R, Fausa O, Lundell L. Omeprazole or ranitidine in the treatment of reflux esophagitis? *Scand J Gastroenterol*. 1988;23:625–632.

45. Hetzel DJ, Dent J, Reed WJ, et al. Healing and relapse of severe peptic esophagitis after treatment with omeprazole. *Gastroenterology.* 1988;95:903–912.

46. Castell DO, Richter JE, Robinson M, et al. Efficacy and safety of lansoprazole in the treatment of erosive esophagitis. *Am J Gastroenterol.* 1996;91:1749–1757.

47. Vigneri S, Termini R, Leandro G, et al. A comparison of five maintenance therapies for reflux esophagitis. *N Engl J Med.* 1995;333:1106–1110.

48. Klinkenberg-Knol EC, Festen H, Jansen JB, et al. Long-term treatment with omeprazole for refractory esophagitis: efficacy and safety. *Ann Intern Med.* 1994;121:161–167.

49. Klinkenberg-Knol EC. Eleven years' experience of continuous maintenance treatment with omeprazole in GERD patients. *Gastroenterology.* 1991;98:114. Abstract 180.

50. Kuo B, Castell DO. Optimal dosing of omeprazole 40 mg daily: effects on gastric and esophageal pH and serum gastrin in healthy controls. *Am J Gastroenterol.* 1996;91:1532–1538.

51. Hatlebakk JG, Katz PO, Kuo B, Castell DO. Nocturnal gastric acid breakthrough with omeprazole 40 mg daily: does dosing schedule make a difference? *Gastroenterology.* 1998;114:591.

52. Hatlebakk JG, Katz PO, Castell DO. Proton pump inhibitors should be taken with meals for optimal control of gastric acidity. *Gastroenterology.* 1998;114:592.

53. Peghini PL, Katz PO, Bracy NA, Castell DO. Nocturnal recovery of gastric acid secretion with twice-daily dosing of proton pump inhibitors. *Am J Gastroenterol.* 1998;93:763–767.

54. Peghini PL, Katz PO, Castell DO. Ranitidine controls nocturnal gastric acid breakthrough on omeprazole: a controlled study in normal subjects. *Gastroenterology.* 1998;115:1335–1339.

55. Zimmerman A, Walters JK, Katona B, Souney P. Alternative methods of proton pump inhibitor administration. *Consult Pharmac.* 1986;19:990–998.

56. Kamel PL, Hanson D, Kahrilas PJ. Omeprazole for the treatment of posterior laryngitis. *Am J Med.* 1994;96:321–326.

57. Belafsky PC, Postma GN, Koufman JA. Laryngopharyngeal reflux symptoms improve before changes in physical findings. *Laryngoscope.* 2001;111:979–981.

58. Kuipers EJ, Lundell L, Klinkenberg-Knol EC, et al. Atrophic gastritis and *Helicobacter pylori* infection in patients with reflux esophagitis treated with omeprazole or fundoplication. *N Engl J Med.* 1996;334:1018–1022.

59. Food and Drug Administration. Proton pump inhibitor relabeling for cancer risk not warranted. *FDA Reports.* Nov. 11, 1996.

60. Sheen E, Traidafilopoulos G. Adverse effects of long-term proton pump inhibitor therapy. *Dig Dis Sci.* 2011;56:931–950.

61. Lodato F, Azzaroli F, Turco L, et al. Adverse effects of proton pump inhibitors. *Best Pract Res Clin Gastroenterol.* 2010; 24:193–201.

62. Bavishi C, Dupont HL. Systematic review: the use of proton pump inhibitors and increased susceptibility to enteric infection. *Aliment Pharmacol Ther.* 2011;34:1269–1281.

63. Eom CS, Jeon CY, Lim JW, et al. Use of acid-suppressive drugs and risk of pneumonia: a systematic review and meta-analysis. *CMAJ.* 2011;183:310–319.

64. Johnstone J, Nerenberg K, Loeb M. Meta-analysis: proton pump inhibitor use and the risk of community-acquired pneumonia. *Aliment Pharmacol Ther.* 2010;31:1165–1177.

65. Targownik LE, Lix LM, Leung S, et al. Proton-pump inhibitor use is not associated with osteoporosis or accelerated bone mineral density loss. *Gastroenterology.* 2010;138:8896–8904.

66. Corley DA, Kubo A, Zhao W, et al. Proton pump inhibitors and histamine-2 receptor antagonists are associated with hip fractures among at-risk patients. *Gastroenterology.* 2010;139:93–101.

67. Ngamreungphong S, Leonatiadis GI, Radhi S, et al. Proton pump inhibitors and risk of fracture: a systematic review and meta-analysis of observational studies. *Am J Gastroenterol.* 2011;106:1209–1218; quiz 1219.

68. Targownik LE, Leslie WD, Davison KS, et al. The relationship between proton pump inhibitor use and longitudinal change in bone mineral density: a population-based study from the Canadian Multicentre Osteoporosis Study (CaMos). *Am J Gastroenterol.* 2012;107:1361–1369.

69. Gerson LB, McMahon D, Olkin I, et al. Lack of significant interactions between clopidogrel and proton pump inhibitor therapy: meta-analysis of existing literature. *Dig Dis Sci.* 2012;57:1304–1313.

70. Kwok CS, Jeevanantham V, Dawn B, Loke YK. No consistent evidence of differential cardiovascular risk amongst proton-pump inhibitors when used with clopidogrel: meta-analysis. *Int J Cardiol.* 2012. (Epub ahead of print.) Retrieved February 15, 2013 from http://www.ncbi.nlm.nih.gov/pubmed/22464478

71. Ford GA, Oliver PS, Prior JS, et al. Omeprazole in the treatment of asthmatics with nocturnal symptoms and gastro-oesophageal reflux: a placebo-controlled cross-over study. *Postgrad Med J.* 1994:70:350–354.

72. Meier JH, McNally PR, Punja M, et al. Does omeprazole (Prilosec) improve respiratory function in asthmatics with gastroesophageal reflux? *Dig Dis Sci.* 1994;39:2127–2133.

73. Boeree MJ, Peters FT, Postma DS, Kleinberbeuker JH. Effect of high-dose omeprazole on airway hyperresponsiveness and pulmonary function in patients with obstructive lung disease. *Gastroenterology.* 1995;108:A61.

74. Klinkenberg-Knol EC, Meuwissen SG. Combined gastric and oesophageal 24-hr monitoring and oesophageal manometry in patients with reflux disease, resistant to treatment with omeprazole. *Aliment Pharmacol Ther.* 1990;4:485–490.

75. Harding SM, Richter JE, Guzzo MR, et al. Asthma and gastroesophageal reflux: acid suppression therapy improves asthma outcome. *Am J Med.* 1996;100:395–405.

76. Hanson DG, Kamel PL, Kahrilas PJ. Outcomes of antireflux therapy for the treatment of chronic laryngitis. *Ann Otol Rhinol Laryngol.* 1995;104:550–555.

77. Wo JM, Grist WJ, Gussack G, et al. Empiric trial of high dose omeprazole in patients with posterior laryngitis. *Am J Gastroenterol.* 1997;92:2160–2165.

78. Metz DC, Childs ML, Ruiz C, Weinstein GS. Pilot study of the oral omeprazole test for reflux laryngitis. *Otolaryngol Head Neck Surg.* 1997;116:41–46.

79. Jaspersen D, Weber R, Hammar CH, Draf W. Effect of omeprazole for the treatment of reflux associated chronic laryngitis. *J Gastroenterology.* 1996;31:765–767.

80. El-Serag HB, Sonnenberg A. Comorbid occurrence of laryngeal or pulmonary disease with esophagitis in United States military veterans. *Gastroenterology.* 1997;113:755–760.

81. El-Serag HB, Lee P, Buchner A, et al. Lansoprazole treatment of patients with chronic idiopathic laryngitis: a placebo-controlled trial. *Am J Gastroenterol.* 2001;96:979–983.

82. Noordzij J, Khidir A, Evans BA, et al. Evaluation of omeprazole in the treatment of reflux laryngitis: a prospective, placebo-controlled, randomized, double-blind study. *Laryngoscope.* 2001;111:2147–2151.

83. Eherer AJ, Habermann W, Hammer HF, et al. Effect of pantoprazole on the course of reflux-associated laryngitis: a placebo-controlled double-blind crossover study. *Scand J Gastroenterol.* 2003;38:462–467.

84. Issing WJ, Tauber S, Folwaczny C, et al. Impact of 24-hour intraesophageal pH monitoring with 2 channels in the diagnosis of reflux-induced otolaryngologic disorders [in German]. *Laryngorhinootology.* 2003;82:347–352.

85. Bilgen C, Ogut F, Kesimli-Dinc H, et al. The comparison of an empiric proton pump inhibitor vs 24-hour double-probe pH monitoring in laryngopharyngeal reflux. *J Laryngol Otol.* 2003;117: 386–390.

86. Bruley des Varannes S, Coron E, Galmiche JP. Short and long-term PPI treatment for GERD. Do we need more-potent anti-secretory drugs? *Best Pract Res Clin Gastroenterol.* 2010;24:905–921.

87. Tighe MP, Afzal NA, Bevan A, Beattie RM. Current pharmacological management of gastro-esophageal reflux in children: an evidence-based systematic review. *Paediatr Drugs.* 2009;11:185–202.

88. Romano C, Chiaro A, Comito D, Loddo I, Ferrau V. Proton pump inhibitors in pediatrics: evaluation of efficacy in GERD therapy. *Curr Clin Pharmacol.* 2011;6:41–47.

89. Lam PK, Ng ML, Cheung TK, et al. Rabeprazole is effective in treating laryngopharyngeal reflux in a randomized placebo-controlled trial. *Clin Gastroenterol Hepatol.* 2010;8:770–776.

90. Masaany M, Marina MB, Ezat WP, Sani A. Empirical treatment with pantoprazole as a diagnostic tool for symptomatic adult laryngopharyngeal reflux. *J Laryngol Otol.* 2011;125:502–508.

91. Abou-Ismail A, Vaezi MF. Evaluation of patients with suspected laryngopharyngeal reflux: a practical approach. *Curr Gastroenterol Rep*. 2011;13:213–218.

92. Dadabhai A, Friedenberg FK. Raberprazole: a pharmacologic and clinical review for acid-related disorders. *Expert Opin Drug Saf*. 2009;8:119–126.

93. Fass R, Noelck N, Willis MR, et al. The effect of esomeprazole 20mg twice daily on acoustic and perception parameters of the voice in laryngopharyngeal reflux. *Neurogastroenterol Motil*. 2010;22:134–141, e44–e45.

94. Johnston N, Bulmer D, Gill GA, et al. Cell biology of laryngeal epithelial defenses in health and disease: further studies. *Ann Otol Rhinol Laryngol*. 2003;112:481–491.

95. Reichel O, Dressel H, Wiederänders K, et al. Double-blind, placebo-controlled trial with esomeprazole for symptoms and signs associated with laryngopharyngeal reflux. *Otolaryngol Head Neck Surg*. 2008;139:414–420.

96. Amin MR, Postma GN, Johnson P, et al. Proton pump inhibitor resistance in the treatment of laryngopharyngeal reflux. *Otolaryngol Head Neck Surg*. 2001;125:374–378.

97. Chiverton SG, Howden CW, Burget DW, Hunt RH. Omeprazole (20 mg) daily given in the morning or evening: a comparison of effects on gastric acidity, and plasma gastrin and omeprazole concentration. *Aliment Pharmacol Ther*. 1992;6:103–111.

98. Bough ID Jr, Sataloff RT, Castell DO, et al. Gastroesophageal reflux disease resistant to omeprazole therapy. *J Voice*. 1995;9:205–211.

99. Leite LP, Johnston BT, Just RJ, Castell DO. Persistent acid secretion during omeprazole therapy: a study of gastric acid profiles in patients demonstrating failure of omeprazole therapy. *Am J Gastroenterol*. 1996;91:1527–1531.

100. Belafsky PC, Rees CJ, Rodriguez K, et al. Esophagopharyngeal reflux. *Otolaryngol Head Neck Surg*. 2008; 138:57–61.

101. Goddard A, Logan R. One-week low-dose triple therapy: new standards for *Helicobacter pylori treatment. Eur J Gastroenterol Hepatol*. 1995;7:1–3.

102. Youssef TF, Ahmed MR. Treatment of clinically diagnosed laryngopharyngeal reflux disease. *Arch Otolaryngol Head Neck Surg*. 2010; 136:1089–1092.

103. Cerulli CE, Portnoy JE, Gregory N, Hawkshaw MJ, Sataloff RT. *Efficacy of superdose proton-pump inhibitor administration in refactory laryngopharyngeal reflux: a pilot study*. Presented at The Voice Foundation's 41st Annual Symposium on Care of the Professional Voice; manuscript in preparation.

104. Weber B, Castellanos A, Hawkshaw MJ, Sataloff RT. *Efficacy of antireflux surgery on refactory laryngopharyngeal reflux disease in professional voice users: a pilot study*. Presented at The Voice Foundation's 41st Annual Symposium on Care of the Professional Voice; manuscript in preparation.

105. Anderson C, Katz PO, Khoury R, Castell DO. Distal esophageal reflux accompanies nocturnal gastric acid breakthrough in patients with gastroesophageal reflux disease (GERD) on proton pump inhibitor (PPI) bid. *Gastroenterology*. 1998;114:229.

106. Katzka DA, Paoletti V, Leite L, Castell DO. Prolonged ambulatory pH monitoring in patients with persistent GERD symptoms: testing while on therapy identifies need for more aggressive antireflux therapy *Am J Gastroenterol*. 1996;91:2110–2113.

107. Peghini P, Katz PO, Castell DO. Bedtime ranitidine decreases gastric acid secretion and eliminates acid exposure overnight in a patient with Barrett's esophagus taking omeprazole, 20 mg bid. *Am J Gastroenterol*. 1997;92:1723.

108. Leite L, Johnston BT, Barrett J, et al. Ineffective esophageal motility (IEM): the primary finding in patients with nonspecific esophageal motility disorder. *Dig Dis Sci*. 1997;42:1859–1865.

109. Fouad YM, Khoury R, Hatlebakk JG, Castell DO. Ineffective esophageal motility (IEM) is more prevalent in reflux patients with respiratory symptoms. *Gastroenterology*. 1998;114:506.

110. Belafsky PC, Postma GN, Koufman JA. Laryngopharyngeal reflux symptoms improve before changes in physical findings. *Laryngoscope*. 2001;111:979–981.

111. Reichel O, Keller J, Rasp G, et al. Efficacy of once-daily esomeprazole treatment in patients with laryngopharyngeal reflux evaluated by 24-h pH monitoring. *Otolaryngol Head Neck Surg*. 2007; 136:205–210.

112. Jin BJ, Lee YS, Jeong SW, et al. Change of acoustic parameters before and after treatment in laryngopharyngeal reflux patients. *Laryngoscope*. 2008;118:938–941.

113. Chapman DB, Rees CJ, Lippert D, Sataloff RT, Wright SC Jr. Adverse effects of long-term proton pump inhibitor use: a review for otolaryngologist. *J Voice*. 2011;25:236–240.

114. Sataloff RT. Proton pump inhibitor: adverse effects [Editorial]. *ENT Journal* 2010;89(12):574-576.

115. Davies M, Wilton LV, Shakir SA. Safety profile of esomeprazole: results of a prescription-event monitoring study of 11,595 patients in England. *Drug Saf*. 2008;31:313-23.

116. Yang YX, Lewis JD, Epstein S, Metz DC. Long-term proton pump inhibitor therapy and risk of hip fracture. *JAMA*. 2006;296: 2947–2953.

117. Aseeri M, Schroeder T, Kramer J, Zackula R. Gastric acid suppression by proton pump inhibitors as a risk factor for *Clostridium difficile*-associated diarrhea in hospitalized patients. *Am J Gastroenterol*. 2008;103:2308–2313.

118. Gilard M, Arnaud B, Cornily C, et al. Influence of omeprazole on the antiplatelet action of clopidogrel associated with aspirin: the randomized, double-blind OCLA (Omeprazole Clopidogrel Aspirin) study. *J Am Coll Cardiol*. 2008;51:256–260.

119. Pezalla E, Day D, Pulliadath I. Initial assessment of clinical impact of a drug interaction between clopidogrel and proton pump inhibitors. *J Am Coll Cardiol*. 2008;52:1038–1039.

120. Eslami L, Kalantarian S, Nasseri-Moghaddam S, Majdzadeh R. Long-term proton pump inhibitor (PPI) use and the incidence of gastric (pre)malignant lesions. *Cochrane Database Syst Rev*. 2008; CD007098.

121. Freston JW. Omeprazole, hypergastrinemia, and gastric carcinoid tumors. *Ann Intern Med*. 1994;121:232–233.

122. Reimer C, Sendergaard B, Hilsted L, Bytzer P. Proton-pump inhibitor therapy induces acid-related symptoms in healthy volunteers after withdrawal of therapy. *Gastroenterology*. 2009;137:80–87.

9

Surgical Therapy for Gastroesophageal Reflux Disease

HISTORICAL OVERVIEW

The history of surgical therapy for the treatment of gastroesophageal reflux began with the work of Phillip Allison, who was the first to correlate the symptoms of hiatal hernia with gastroesophageal reflux.[1] His repair, described in 1951, emphasized the need to place the gastroesophageal junction intra-abdominally to improve its function. This maneuver alone, however, was found to be associated with a high rate of symptom recurrence. More sophisticated attempts at securing the gastroesophageal junction below the diaphragm culminated in the posterior gastropexy described by Hill in 1967.[2] This operation is still in use, although it has largely been replaced by fundoplication.

Rudolph Nissen described his gastric fundus wrap in 1956.[3] His innovations were followed by a flurry of interest in surgical management for this disease. However, over the past 2 decades, surgical treatment for reflux has become much less commonly used, owing to the introduction of more effective agents in medical therapy, specifically histamine-2 (H_2) blockers and proton-pump inhibitors (PPIs).

In 1991, the first reports of laparoscopic antireflux surgery (the Nissen fundoplication) were published.[4] The availability of minimally invasive approaches made surgery more acceptable to gastroenterologists and patients, leading to a resurgence of interest in surgical management of gastroesophageal reflux disease (GERD). Since the initial clinical reports in 1991, numerous studies have been published on the laparoscopic approach to antireflux surgery.[5–18]

Medical therapy is effective in controlling acid reflux in the majority of patients with GERD. However, although usually effective in controlling symptoms, medical therapy does not correct the mechanical abnormality that causes reflux. Patients often require long-term or indefinite courses of medications, as discontinuation frequently leads to recurrence of symptoms. In a series of 196 patients with severe esophagitis responsive to omeprazole, 82% developed recurrent erosions within 6 months after cessation of therapy.[19] Moreover, the consequences of long-term acid suppression are unknown.

In 1992, Spechler[20] compared the outcomes with medical versus surgical therapy for complicated GERD. Surgery was significantly more effective, resulting in greater patient satisfaction, increased lower esophageal sphincter (LES) pressures, lesser grades of esophagitis, and lower levels of esophageal acid exposure. This study had an average 2-year follow-up but was done without the use of PPIs.

However, in a follow-up study in 2001, Spechler et al[21] found no significant long-term differences between the groups in terms of grade of esophagitis, frequency of treatment of esophageal stricture and subsequent antireflux operations, SF-36 standardized physical and mental component scale scores, and overall satisfaction with antireflux therapy. They suggested that antireflux surgery should not be advised with the expectation that patients with GERD will no longer need to take antisecretory medications or that the procedure will prevent esophageal cancer among those with GERD and Barrett's esophagus. So et al[22] compared laparoscopic fundoplication results in patients complaining of atypical symptoms with results in patients who had typical GERD symptoms (heartburn and regurgitation). They found that postoperative relief of atypical symptoms was less satisfactory and more difficult to predict than relief of heartburn and regurgitation. The only predictors of relief of atypical symptoms were preoperative response to pharmacologic acid suppression and dual-probe pH testing (only in patients with laryngeal symptoms). Preoperative relief of atypical symptoms with use of a PPI or an H_2 blocker was significantly associated with successful surgical outcome. Findings of other authors who have assessed the effects of antireflux surgery on atypical symptoms have been variable.[23–28] For example, Larrain et al[26] found that antireflux surgery produced symptomatic improvement in GERD-related asthma and reduced the need for bronchodilators. However, Pitcher et al[28] found that antireflux surgery did not reliably relieve reflux-related asthma. In 1996, Hunter et al[29] reported atypical symptom improvement rates of 80% to 91% in patients undergoing laparoscopic fundoplication, with particularly good results in the subset of patients with laryngopharyngeal symptoms. Although the role of antireflux surgery remains controversial, in our experience it has proved valuable in appropriately selected voice patients.

INDICATIONS FOR SURGICAL THERAPY

Indications for surgery include persistent symptomatology despite reasonable medical management and patient intolerance to medications. Surgery may also be an option for patients who are concerned about the costs and consequences of long-term medical therapy. In patients whose symptom control requires continuous medical therapy, surgery is an important option. Patients with complicated GERD, who manifest Barrett's metaplasia, stricture, or ulceration, and who require long-term therapy should also be considered for surgery.

In the past, surgery for GERD was recommended infrequently owing to the risks associated with abdominal surgery conducted with the patient under general anesthesia, significant postoperative discomfort, and the recognition of substantial long-term complications such as dysphagia, "gas bloat," and others. Since its initial description by Rudolph Nissen in 1956, the operation has undergone significant modifications that have lessened the incidence of postoperative complications.[30] In addition, with the introduction of the laparoscopic approach to antireflux surgery, the postoperative discomfort, as well as many of the risks, has been minimized. The laparoscopic approach has also shortened the postoperative recuperation period from 6 to 8 weeks to 2 to 3 weeks, allowing patients to return to normal activities in an acceptable period of time.

PREOPERATIVE EVALUATION

Thorough preoperative evaluation is essential to successful surgical management of GERD. Although the typical patient with this disorder has well-recognized gastrointestinal (GI) symptoms, in certain cases GERD may underlie asthma and other respiratory diseases, laryngitis, chronic cough, and chest pain. In addition, patients with other upper GI conditions may present with symptoms similar to those seen with GERD. Thus, it is critical to firmly establish the diagnosis and to exclude other conditions.

Further goals of preoperative evaluation are to assess the anatomy and physiology of the swallowing mechanism and stomach. Adequacy of esophageal motility and of gastric emptying are important preoperative considerations, as disorders in either of these areas will affect the choice of a surgical procedure. It is also important to document complications of reflux, specifically the presence or absence of Barrett's metaplasia, ulceration, or stricture.

The preoperative evaluation should include the following:

1. A complete history and physical examination is especially important both to identify symptoms related to reflux and to exclude other conditions. Evaluation of the general medical status is also crucial.
2. Upper gastrointestinal endoscopy is important to exclude other lesions and to assess for the presence or absence of Barrett's metaplasia. Stricture and ulceration may also be seen. The presence or absence of *Helicobacter pylori* may be determined.
3. Roentgenographic barium contrast study of the upper GI tract defines the anatomy of the esophagus and stomach, as well as the

relationship of the gastroesophageal junction to the hiatus. The length of the esophagus is assessed easily; the presence of a foreshortened esophagus alters surgical management significantly, as discussed later on. The presence of a sliding or paraesophageal hernia can be determined. In addition, other anatomic abnormalities of the esophagus and stomach can be identified, such as strictures, webs, masses, or diverticula. Furthermore, this is a dynamic study, allowing the radiologist to assess the motility of the esophagus and the emptying function of the stomach. Although reflux of barium is not always identified, the absence of this finding does not rule out the presence of reflux; demonstration of significant reflux of barium during this radiographic procedure is almost always considered abnormal. An assessment of gastric emptying also can be performed. This information can be obtained from the upper GI series or from a gastric emptying study. It is important to document the status of gastric emptying prior to surgical intervention that occurs in the area of the vagal trunks, as there have been occasional reports of postoperative gastroparesis.

4. Twenty-four-hour pH monitoring is considered the most accurate test for documenting the presence of abnormal acid reflux. This study is particularly useful in patients who present with atypical symptoms such as asthma, chronic cough, hoarseness, and chest pain. This study quantifies the amount of abnormal reflux, defines its relationship to symptomatology, assesses for its presence in upright or supine positions, and evaluates the relationship of reflux episodes to time of day and specific activities. Although this study is not strictly obligatory in patients with typical symptoms of reflux and evidence of reflux obtained by other means (eg, endoscopic evidence of ulcerative esophagitis or Barrett's metaplasia), it is a useful baseline to help assess postoperative results objectively.

5. Esophageal manometry is obligatory in the preoperative evaluation of the patient with GERD. This essential study provides information regarding LES pressure, length, and relaxation. It also provides vital information regarding esophageal motility. Major motility abnormalities of the esophagus alter the choice of surgical procedure.

6. Other studies and evaluations include pulmonary function testing and comprehensive voice evaluations in selected patients. These studies are particularly valuable in patients presenting with atypical symptoms.

PATHOPHYSIOLOGY OF GASTROESOPHAGEAL REFLUX DISEASE AND SURGICAL CORRECTION

GERD results from a loss of competence of the antireflux barrier at the gastroesophageal junction. Improper functioning of the gastroesophageal junction can be due to multiple factors, including transient inappropriate relaxations of the LES, primary hypotension of the LES, shortened LES length, shortened intra-abdominal segment of the LES, loss of a flap valve, delayed gastric emptying, and abnormalities in esophageal clearance, among others.[31] Incompetence of the gastroesophageal junction is a mechanical defect that is amenable to surgical correction. To maximize competence at the gastroesophageal junction and to minimize postsurgical complications, the proper antireflux operation should include the following:

- Mobilization of the esophagus to restore intra-abdominal length
- Correction of the diaphragmatic defect
- The creation of a short, loose fundoplication around the distal esophagus just proximal to the gastroesophageal junction anchored to the esophagus for stability.

CURRENT OPERATIVE PROCEDURES FOR CORRECTION OF GASTROESOPHAGEAL REFLUX DISEASE

Antireflux procedures can be classified into 2 groups: those that involve some form of fundoplication and those that do not. They can also be classified by surgical approach, specifically, whether the procedure is performed through the abdomen or through the chest.[32] Additionally, all these operations can be done as open procedures or using minimally invasive techniques (laparoscopic and thoracoscopic approaches).

In selecting an antireflux operation, all preoperative information needs to be considered. Esophageal function and motility affect the choice of operation. When motility is normal, the Nissen fundoplication with a full 360-degree wrap is the operation of choice. Conversely, with major motility abnormalities, a partial fundoplication is usually preferable.

Second, the length of the esophagus is important. Esophageal shortening should be corrected with the addition of a gastroplasty. Third, the presence or absence of hypersecretions of gastric acid may play a role in choice of surgical procedure. An acid-reducing procedure such as a selective vagotomy may be considered in addition to the antireflux procedure. Fourth, the finding of a significant gastroparesis preoperatively may prompt consideration of an additional gastric procedure such as a pyloroplasty at the time of antireflux repair.

SURGICAL REPAIRS INVOLVING NISSEN FUNDOPLICATION

In 1956, Rudolph Nissen described his 360-degree gastric fundic wrap.[3] Since that time, modifications regarding the length and looseness of the wrap have been made, allowing the most effective antireflux procedure with minimal morbidity. Currently, this is the most popular antireflux procedure. The steps in performing fundoplication, which are similar whether the approach is open or laparoscopic, include the following:

1. Incision of the gastrohepatic omentum at the gastroesophageal junction to expose the esophagus and the diaphragmatic crura (Figures 9–1 and 9–2)

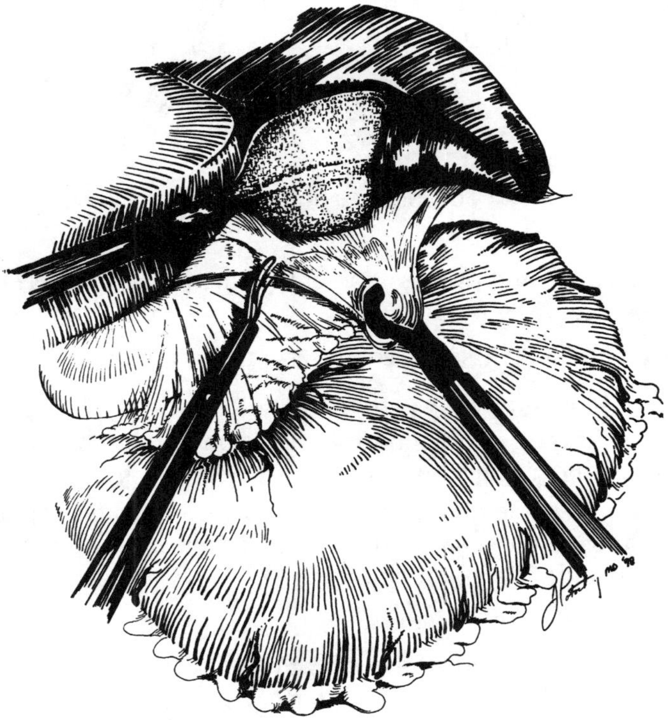

Figure 9–1. Incision of gastrohepatic omentum.

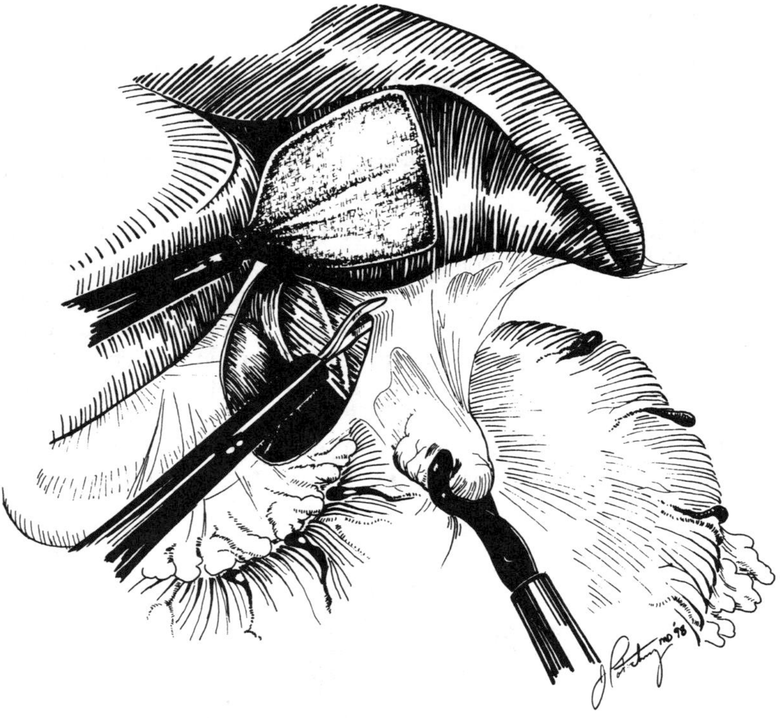

Figure 9–2. Exposure of esophagus and diaphragmatic crura.

2. Identification and preservation of the anterior and posterior vagus nerves (Figure 9–3)
3. Circumferential dissection of the esophagus (Figure 9–4)
4. Assessment of mobility of the fundus
   a. Mobilization of the fundus by division of the short gastric vessels if the fundus is not sufficiently floppy (Figure 9–5)
   b. With a sufficiently floppy fundus, occasional omission of mobilization of the short gastric vessels, creating a Rossetti modification of the Nissen fundoplication
5. Closure of the crura (Figure 9–6)
6. Construction of a loose fundoplication around the distal esophagus just proximal to the gastroesophageal junction. This maneuver is performed over a large (54F–56F) dilator, and the fundic wrap created is 2 cm in length (Figure 9–7).

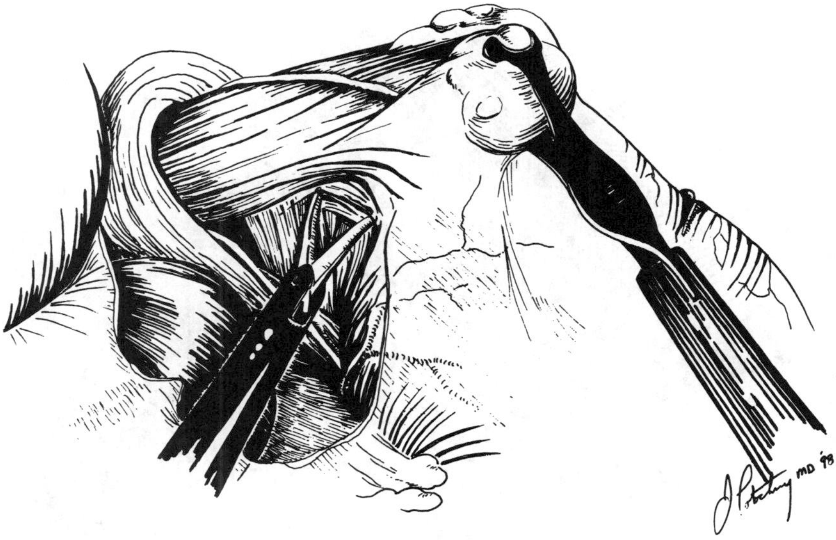

Figure 9–3. Identification of vagus nerves.

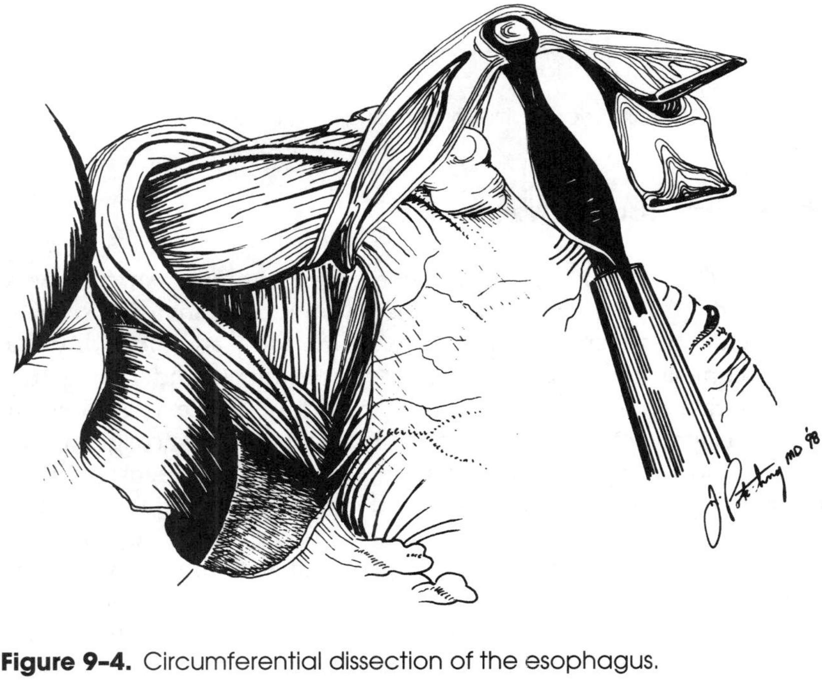

Figure 9–4. Circumferential dissection of the esophagus.

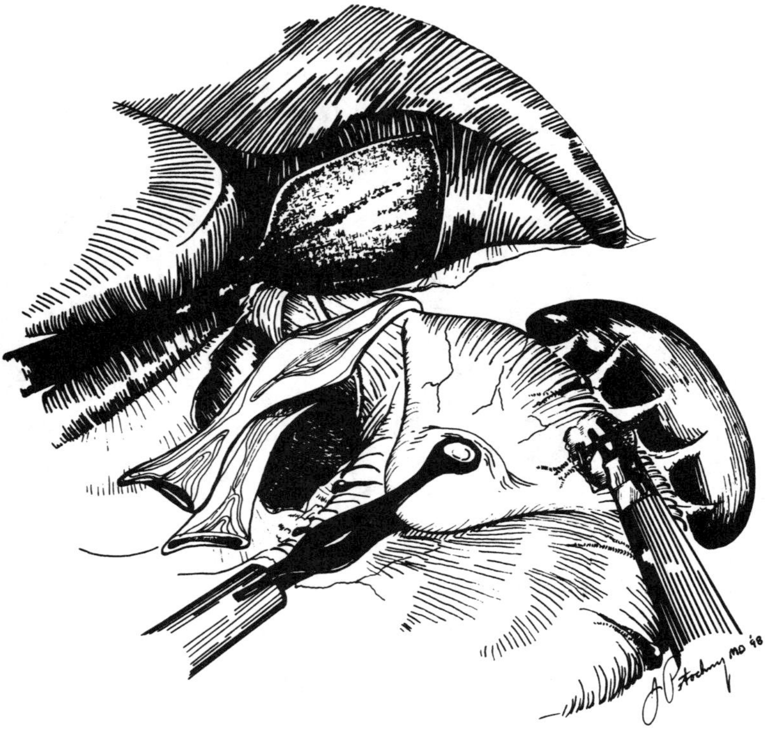

Figure 9-5. Mobilization of the proximal greater curvature.

The Laparoscopic Approach

In the 1990s, the first reports of laparoscopic antireflux surgery were published.[4–18] These reports described a minimally invasive surgical approach to treatment of GERD with low mortality and morbidity. The laparoscopic approach can be used in most patients undergoing antireflux surgery and has become the approach of choice. Contraindications to a laparoscopic antireflux operation include major coagulopathy, severe obstructive pulmonary disease, and possibly pregnancy. Prior abdominal surgery is not a contraindication. Reoperative antireflux surgery usually cannot be performed laparoscopically. Occasionally, a laparoscopic approach may be attempted, but generally, conversion to an open procedure has been necessary. The reason for conversion is usually severe central obesity or a large left lobe of the liver, both of which preclude adequate visualization of the relevant anatomy.

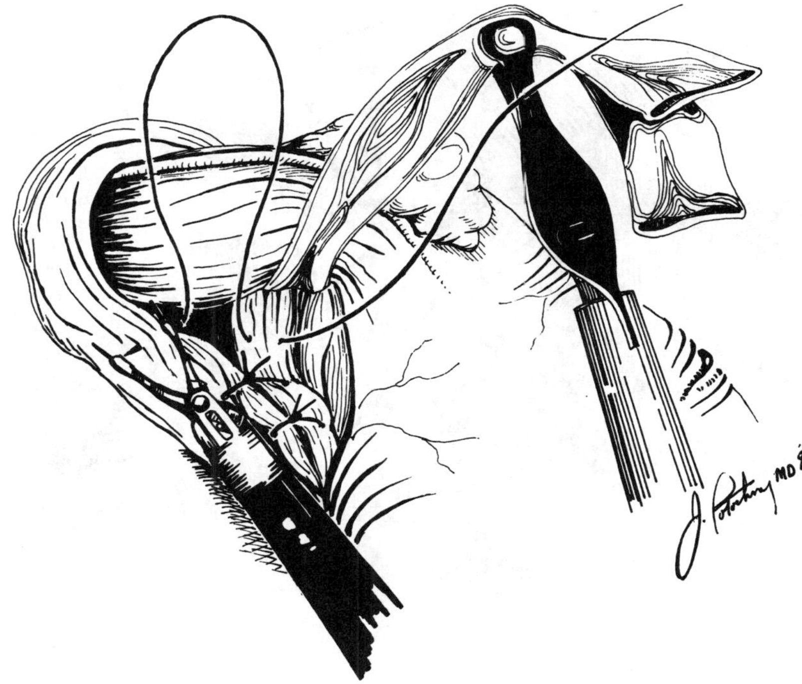

Figure 9–6. Closure of the crura.

The patient is placed on the operating table in a combined lithotomy and reverse Trendelenburg position. This positioning allows the surgeon to be stationed between the patient's legs, which facilitates the 2-handed dissection essential to satisfactory performance of the procedure. However, the 2-handed technique also can be used effectively with the patient in the supine position, with the surgeon situated on the left side of the table and port placement modified somewhat (Figure 9–8).

A 12-mm port is positioned to the right of the xiphoid for the liver retractor. Right upper quadrant and left upper quadrant 10-mm ports are placed to function as dissecting ports. An additional 10-mm port in the midline is used for placement of the camera, and a 10-mm port is placed in the left midabdomen for retraction of the stomach. The left lobe of the liver is retracted upward, exposing the gastroesophageal junction. A laparoscopic Babcock clamp is used to pull down the fundus, exposing the hiatus.

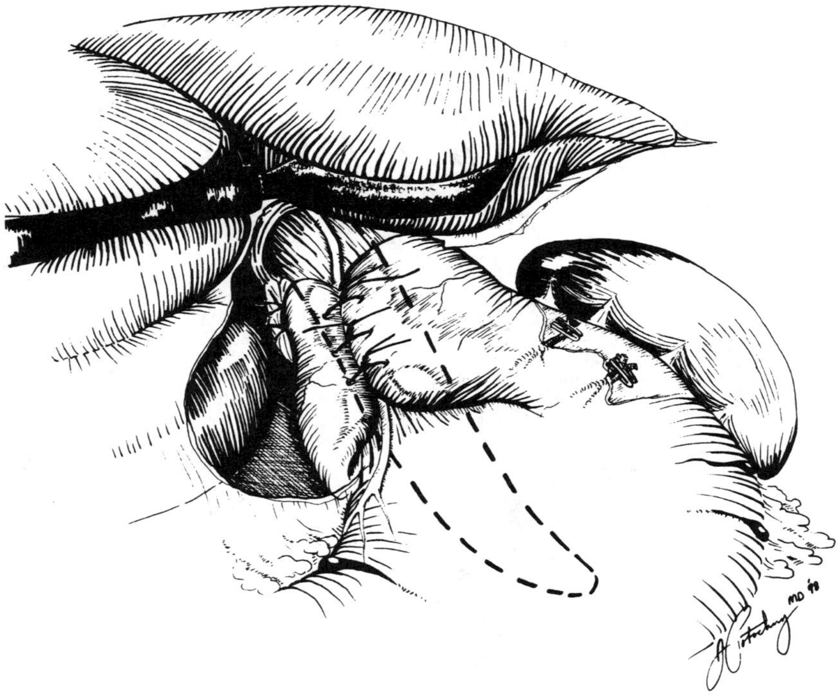

Figure 9–7. Construction of fundoplication.

The gastrohepatic omentum overlying the gastroesophageal junction is incised, and the right crus is identified. The right crus is dissected away from the right lateral wall of the esophagus, and the left crus is identified and dissected away from the left side of the esophagus. The esophagus is then retracted upward, and the posterior aspect of the esophagus is dissected under direct vision. It is important to perform the esophageal dissection under direct vision at all times to avoid perforation. Furthermore, dissection should not stray from the esophagus, as dissection in the pleural space can occur, causing pneumothorax. Once the esophagus is circumferentially dissected, a Penrose drain is placed around it, and the Babcock clamp previously used to retract the fundus is repositioned on the Penrose drain. The anterior (left) and posterior (right) vagus nerves are identified. The posterior nerve is excluded from the Penrose drain.

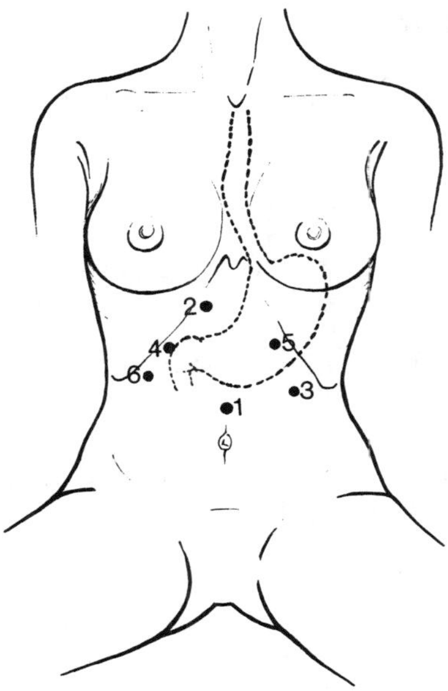

Figure 9–8. Port placement for laparoscopic fundoplication:
1. 30-degree laparoscope
2. Liver retractor
3. Stomach retractor
4. Dissecting port
5. Dissecting port
6. Optional dissecting port

The fundus is then inspected to assess its mobility. In most cases, it is advisable to divide the short gastric vessels to allow for a loose, tension-free wrap. Division can be accomplished using the harmonic scalpel or clips. The proximal third of the greater curvature is mobilized in this manner.

The diaphragmatic opening is made appropriately snug. This step is performed with a 54F–56F dilator within the esophagus to avoid making the closure too tight. Once the diaphragmatic closure is completed, the dilator is retracted into the midesophagus by the anesthesiologist or an assistant. The fundus is then drawn around the posterior surface of the esophagus. The wrap is accomplished over the 54F–56F dilator by placing three 2-0 silk sutures. These sutures are placed from the fundus to the esophagus to the other side of the fundus in each instance. The abdomen is then irrigated, and hemostasis is ensured. All trocars are removed under direct vision, and port sites are closed.

The Transthoracic Approach

Indications for performing an antireflux procedure via the thorax are as follows:

- Reoperative antireflux surgery
- The need for a concomitant procedure on the intrathoracic esophagus
- Coexistent left pulmonary pathology that necessitates surgery
- Presence of a foreshortened esophagus
- Presence of obesity severe enough to affect visualization with an abdominal approach
- Surgeon preference.

Partial Fundoplication

In the presence of esophageal dysmotility, partial fundoplication is the operation of choice. This can be performed through a thoracic approach such as a Belsey Mark IV partial fundoplication, which creates a 240-degree anterior partial fundoplication. Alternatively, the Toupet partial fundoplication can be performed transabdominally as an open or a laparoscopic procedure. The technical aspects of this procedure are similar to those for a Nissen fundoplication, with the exception of the wrap. After mobilization of the fundus and pulling it around posterior to the esophagus, the fundus is sutured to the right crus using three 2-0 silk sutures.

The anterior aspect of the fundus is then sutured to the esophagus. The fundus is similarly sutured to the left crus and anteriorly along the left side of the esophagus. This wrap necessitates placement of 12 sutures in the 4 rows (Figure 9–9).

Collis Gastroplasty

In patients with a foreshortened esophagus, a Collis gastroplasty is utilized to lengthen the esophagus. This is followed by a partial or complete fundoplication around the gastric tube with placement of the repair intra-abdominally (Figure 9–10).

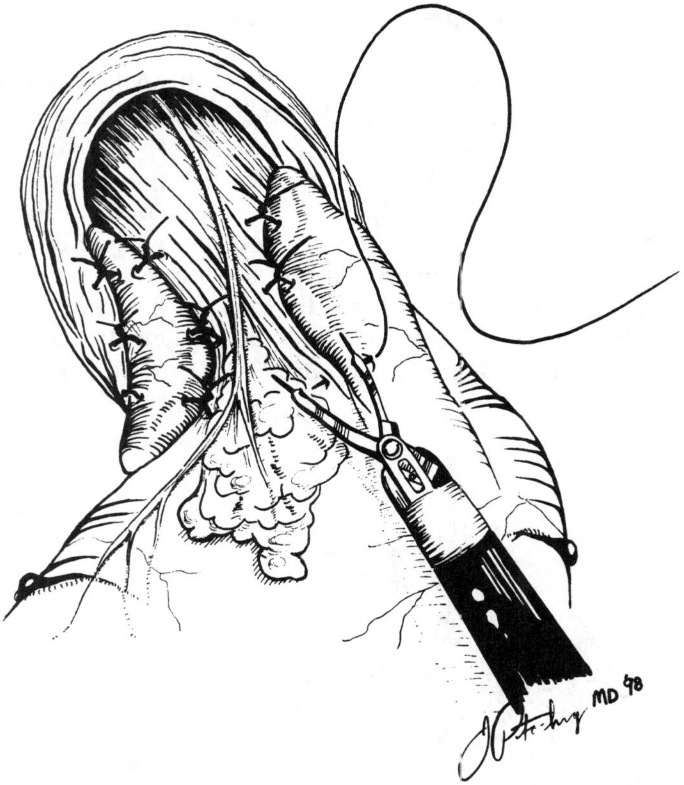

Figure 9–9. Partial fundoplication (Toupet).

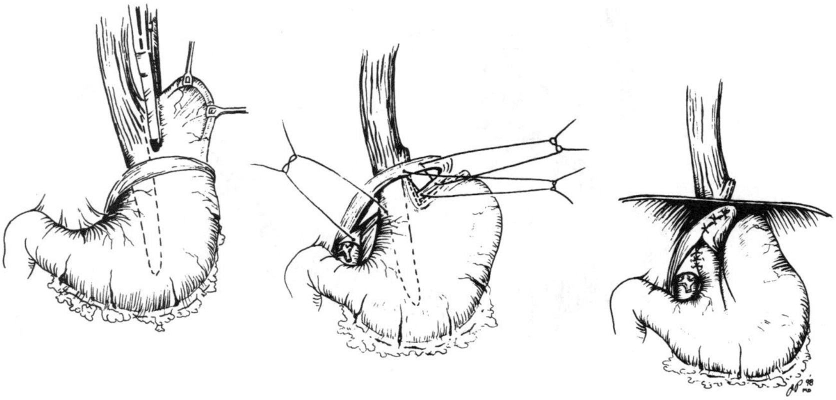

Figure 9–10. Collis gastroplasty.

NONFUNDOPLICATION REPAIRS (GASTROPEXY)

In 1967, Lucius Hill[2] described his experience with posterior gastropexy. After his initial series, approximately 20% of his patients experienced recurrence of reflux symptoms on long-term follow-up. This result led to modifications of the technique to include calibration of the LES pressure performed intraoperatively. The physiologic basis of the current Hill operation is restoration of the LES segment to the high-pressure environment of the abdomen, where it is secured by anchoring the gastroesophageal junction to the median arcuate ligament posteriorly. The hiatal hernia defect is corrected, and the LES pressure is reassessed using intraoperative manometry (Figure 9–11). The Hill repair has been

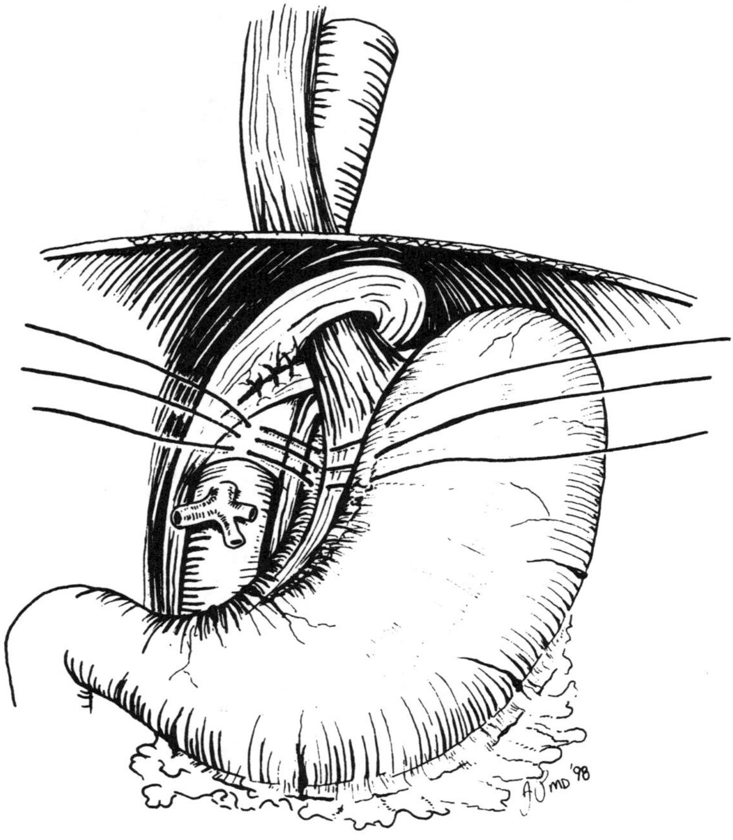

Figure 9–11. Hill posterior gastropexy.

described utilizing an open or laparoscopic technique.[33] The following steps are common to both:

1. The crura are dissected.
2. The anterior and posterior vagus nerves are identified and preserved.
3. The esophagus is dissected circumferentially.
4. The medial aspect of the gastric fundus is mobilized from its adhesions to the diaphragm, which occasionally also includes division of several short gastric vessels.
5. The preaortic fascia is dissected down to the area of the median arcuate ligament.
6. The esophageal hiatus is loosely closed around the esophagus.
7. Sutures are placed in the anterior and posterior phrenoesophageal bundles, with care taken to avoid the esophagus. Three such sutures are placed.
8. Intraoperative manometry is performed. Sutures are placed through the imbricated bundles and carried through the preaortic fascia.
9. Additional sutures are placed from the fundus through the diaphragm to further reinforce the gastroesophageal valve.

POSTOPERATIVE CARE

The patient is admitted to the hospital postoperatively. A nasogastric tube is not used routinely. Antireflux medications are not restarted. On the first postoperative day, the patient undergoes an upper GI contrast study using a water-soluble contrast agent to rule out the presence of a leak. If no leak is identified, the patient is asked to swallow a small amount of barium to delineate more fully the postoperative anatomy and to assess emptying function of the esophagus and stomach. Clear liquids are started on the first postoperative day, and the diet is advanced as tolerated. With laparoscopic surgery, the patient is generally discharged on the second postoperative day. Some degree of minor transient dysphagia is common, but in nearly all cases this problem resolves within 8 to 12 weeks.

Patients are seen for follow-up evaluation at 2 weeks postoperatively. At 3 and 12 months, patients are asked to undergo repeat 24-hour pH monitoring and esophageal manometry.

OPERATIVE COMPLICATIONS

In general, antireflux surgery, whether performed open or closed, is safe. In several large series, mortality rates were essentially zero.[12,14] Wound complications such as infection and herniation are seen slightly more often with the open technique. In addition, splenic injury is reported to occur in 1% to 2% of open fundoplications, but it is very rarely, if ever, seen with the laparoscopic approach. Idani et al[34] suggested that the success of fundoplication and prevention of postoperative complications including dysphagia often depend on surgical technique. The authors suggest that the gastric fundus be lifted up toward the cranium without being twisted, with the anterior and posterior walls of the fundus forming the left and right sides, respectively, of the fundoplication. Kosek et al[35] reported that division of the short gastric vessels during laparoscopic Nissen fundoplication remains controversial. In their patients, routine division of the short gastric vessels did not result in functional or clinical damage during short-term or long-term follow-up.

Esophageal transit and gastric emptying scores can aid in evaluation of surgical outcome following laparoscopic fundoplication. Schuchert and colleagues[36] reported no significant differences in pre- and postoperative esophageal transit and gastric emptying scores in their patients following fundoplication.

Complications following laparoscopic antireflux surgery include those common to all operations, those specific to laparoscopy, and those related to the specific surgical procedure. Operative complications common to all procedures include bleeding and infection. Bleeding complications are rarely, if ever, seen with laparoscopic antireflux surgery. Blood transfusions are virtually never necessary. Wound infection is also extremely uncommon. Another complication common to many operations performed under general anesthesia is pulmonary embolism. In our series of 70 laparoscopic antireflux procedures, this complication occurred in 2.8% of patients. In no instance was it fatal.[16]

Complications specific to laparoscopy include trocar injuries, hypercapnea requiring ventilation, pneumothorax, and pneumomediastinum. Trocar injures are rare. We use an open technique for inserting the initial trocar and have not noted any injuries. Many patients have pneumothorax. As part of the original protocol used by one of us (D.M.S.), all patients underwent routine chest x-ray examination in the recovery room, and this finding was incidentally noted commonly. In all instances, patients were asymptomatic, and the pneumothorax resolved on follow-up chest x-ray examination the next day. In addition, pneumomediastinum with occasional tracking of air into the subcutaneous tissues of the neck and chest was seen. In all instances, these abnormalities resolved within 24 hours.

Complications specific to the operation include persistent dysphagia, defined as dysphagia still present more than 3 months after surgery. In the literature, patients have required reoperation for this complication, although we have not had that experience in our series to date. Occasionally, persistent dysphagia can be corrected with endoscopic dilatation. Postoperative gastroparesis is occasionally seen and is thought to be due to edema around the vagus nerves secondary to the operative dissection. This complication is rare and is effectively treated with prokinetic agents such as cisapride and metoclopramide. This phenomenon is generally transient, and these medications can be discontinued several weeks after surgery.

Esophageal or gastric perforation occurring intraoperatively has also been described. Should these complications be recognized intraoperatively, they can be repaired laparoscopically. Such repair requires an experienced surgeon well versed in advanced laparoscopic techniques. Failure to recognize these complications may allow progression to sepsis, which frequently necessitates a return to the operating room. Fortunately, such cases are also rare.

RESULTS

Many studies report the efficacy of antireflux surgery, with 90% of patients demonstrating symptom control. The laparoscopic approach achieves outcomes similar to those obtained with open antireflux surgery, although follow-up to date is shorter.

Professional voice users often experience reflux during singing. This reflux may be acidic or pH neutral. In this subgroup, patients do well following antireflux surgery, with improved vocal quality and strength, although some will still require antireflux medication, at least occasionally.

ENDOSCOPIC ANTIREFLUX THERAPY

Although medical and surgical therapies for GERD are extremely successful, well-studied, and effective alternatives for patients with need for long-term therapy, many patients would prefer a nonsurgical, nonpharmacologic option for treatment of their symptoms. This has led to extensive research and development of endoscopic procedures designed to treat GERD. Four of these procedures are approved by the Food and Drug Administration (FDA) for treatment of GERD: radiofrequency energy delivery to the gastroesophageal junction (Stretta, Curon Medical, Fremont, CA), transoral flexible endoscopic suturing (EndoCinch, Bard, Murray Hill, NJ), injection of a biocompatible, nonbiodegradable copolymer to reinforce the muscular layer of the LES (Enteryx, Boston Scientific, Natick, MA), and an endoscopic, full-thickness plicator device (Ndo plicator). All attempt to reduce reflux by mechanically altering the LES. The exact mechanism for their efficacy is unknown.

Several key generalizations can be made. To date, a relatively small number of patients have been studied, follow-up time is relatively short (≤3 years), and a few major side effects have been reported. Studies have been performed in patients with heartburn and regurgitation.

All patients treated have had good response to PPIs. Only patients with mild erosive esophagitis (grade 2 or less) and small hiatal hernias have been evaluated. Therefore, patients with severe erosive esophagitis, Barrett's esophagus, and other manifestations of GERD (cough, asthma, laryngopharyngeal reflux [LPR]) have not been studied. Although long-term side effects are few, chest pain, dysphagia, and fever are seen immediately after the procedure in most patients. Unfortunately, several deaths have been associated with the procedures (Stretta and Enteryx); other rare major complications such as pleural effusion, esophageal perforation, and aspiration have also been reported.

Stretta

Six months after therapy, patients in an open-label study in the United States who were treated with radiofrequency energy showed an improvement in heartburn score, regurgitation, quality of life, and patient satisfaction compared with baseline without any changes in esophageal motility.[37]

The initial study reported no major complications. At 6 months, 70% were not on any antisecretory therapy and 87% were able to discontinue PPIs. At 1-year follow-up, more than 60% continued to be off antisecretory therapy and had sustained improvement in heartburn. Unfortunately, serious side effects have been reported to the FDA, including aspiration, pleural effusion, atrial fibrillation, and deaths in the first 1000 procedures performed.

Stretta has been studied in a prospective, sham-controlled study.[38] Sixty-four patients were randomly assigned to radiofrequency energy delivery to the gastroesophageal junction (35 patients) or to a sham procedure (29 patients). Radiofrequency energy delivery significantly improved GERD symptoms and quality of life compared with the sham procedure (61% of patients in the treatment group compared with 33% of patients who received a sham procedure ceased to have daily heartburn symptoms), but it did not decrease esophageal acid exposure or medication use at 6 months. Symptom improvement persisted 12 months after treatment, and no perforations or deaths were reported.

EndoCinch

The second approved procedure, endoluminal gastroplication (EndoCinch), was reported initially in a multicenter trial of 64 patients with heartburn more often than 3 times a week, dependence on antisecretory medication, mild erosive esophagitis, and abnormal 24-hour pH monitoring. They were treated with EndoCinch, an endoscopic suturing system designed to create an "internal plication" of the stomach.[39]

In this uncontrolled trial, improvement in the number of reflux episodes was seen. No change in upright, recumbent, or total esophageal acid exposure was seen at 3 and 6 months. Sixty-two percent of patients were able to decrease drugs to <4 doses of antisecretory medications per month. Improvement was seen in patient satisfaction, heartburn severity, and heartburn score compared with the initial measurements. With the exception of a "stitch" perforation that required short-term hospitalization, no major complications were reported. To date, no sham trial has been reported in full manuscript form using this method.

Most recently, a 2-year follow-up study in 33 patients originally treated with this endoscopic device was reported.[40] After a mean follow-up of 25 months, heartburn severity and score and frequency of regurgitation showed continued improvement compared with baseline measurements. However, only 8 patients (25%) initially on PPIs were completely off antisecretory medications, with 9% taking half or less of their initial dose. Forty percent required full dose medications, and 6% had undergone a laparoscopic Nissen fundoplication because of therapeutic failure.

In an open-label, multicenter US trial,[41] 85 patients with GERD were treated with endoluminal gastroplication. At 12 and 24 months postoperatively, 59% and 52%, respectively, showed heartburn symptom resolution, and 73% and 69% decreased their PPI use by at least 50%. Eleven patients had adverse events, only 2 of which were serious: 1 patient had severe dysphagia necessitating removal of the plications, and 1 had severe bronchospasm requiring intubation to allow completion of the procedure. These data are disappointing and suggest that long-term efficacy of this originally designed procedure will not be forthcoming.

Enteryx

The Enteryx procedure was granted approval by the FDA in April 2003. The procedure is performed by injecting a biopolymer (ethylene vinyl alcohol, EVA) into the muscular layer of the LES under fluoroscopic guidance. The proposed mechanism of action is based on enhancing the gastroesophageal barrier against reflux via a space-occupying effect, inducing fibrosis in the area of injection, and altering the compliance of the sphincter during gastric distention.[42]

In the expanded, multicenter, open-label, international clinical trial of Enteryx implantation for GERD,[43] promising results at 12 months and 24 months were reported: 78% and 72%, respectively, of patients were able to reduce their previous PPI dose by at least 50%, and 78% and 80% reported significant improvement of their heartburn-related quality of life symptoms during the same time periods. None of the patients had what was considered a potentially life-threatening adverse event. The most common adverse event was transient retrosternal chest pain in 85% of patients, which resolved with prescription pain medications in 84% of affected patients. One of the 144 enrolled patients developed a paraesophageal fluid collection diagnosed at 6 weeks after the procedure, which resolved completely with intravenous antibiotics.

In a recent randomized, single-blind, prospective, multicenter clinical trial in Europe,[44] 64 patients with classic heartburn symptoms controlled on PPI therapy were randomized into 2 groups of equal sizes to receive either the Enteryx procedure or a sham procedure consisting of a standard upper endoscopy and were followed before allowing for crossover for 3 months. Eighty-one percent of patients in the Enteryx group achieved ≥50% reduction of their PPI use compared with 53% of those in the sham group, and 68% of patients in the Enteryx group versus 41% of patients in the sham group ceased PPIs completely. More Enteryx-treated (81%) than sham-treated (19%) patients did not undergo retreatment. Pain, odynophagia/dysphagia, and fever were the most common adverse events in the Enteryx group. An esophageal ulcer with extrusion of the copolymer was noted in 1 patient. Preliminary results of the US multicenter trial were recently reported with results similar to the European trial. Overall, although pH studies have shown statistical improvement from baseline, normalization is seen in less than one-third of patients.

Although few major side effects have been reported in the organized clinical trials, at least one procedure-related death has been reported, as well as case reports of mediastinitis and pleural effusion.

Endoscopic Full-Thickness Plicator

This system creates a transmural plication 1 cm distal to the esophageal junction, reinforcing the competency of the gastroesophageal barrier. It was granted premarket approval by the FDA in April 2003.

Data on the intermediate-term safety and efficacy of this device were published recently in a multicenter North American trial[45]; 64 patients requiring maintenance antisecretory therapy for chronic heartburn received a single endoscopic full-thickness plication in the gastric cardia 1 cm distal to the gastroesophageal junction. Of the 57 patients who completed the 12-month follow-up by the time of publication, 70% were off PPI therapy. Median heartburn-related quality of life scores improved significantly compared with baseline both while not taking PPIs and while taking such medication. Normal pH scores were observed in 30% of patients. Common procedure-related adverse events included sore throat (41%) and abdominal pain (20%), resolving spontaneously after several days. The same group had reported 6 serious adverse events during the initial follow-up at 6 months[46]: 2 patients experienced severe dyspnea, 1 developed pneumothorax, 1 pneumoperitoneum, 1 gastric perforation, and 1 fundic mucosal abrasion. None resulted in long-term patient injury.

In 2010, Velanovich[47] reported his experience using Esophyx, a device for endoscopic fundoplication. Esophyx was used in 24 patients; 20 had symptoms and signs of GERD and 4 had been diagnosed with LPR. Four of the 24 patients had recurrent symptoms following Nissen procedures. He suggested that much research is still needed and that endoscopic fundoplication is most effective in patients with mild-to-moderate symptoms of GERD and those with small hiatal hernias. Its value for patients with LPR has not been established.

Summary and Role in LPR

The concept of endoscopic therapy is excellent, and its potential is exciting. Nonetheless, we are early in our evaluation of these evolving techniques. No organized clinical trials have been done or are in process in LPR. Therefore, efficacy in these difficult-to-treat patients cannot be predicted. Based on the current outcomes in patients with heartburn, the best that one might expect is the opportunity to reduce PPI dosage. More data on efficacy and safety are needed before we can recommend these techniques widely. Patients should be reminded that medical therapy is safe and surgery a reasonable alternative when performed by an experienced surgeon. Francis et al[48] examined the role of antireflux surgery in patients with signs and symptoms of LPR refractory to medical management with PPIs. They pointed out the controversy regarding the role of fundoplication in patients with PPI-refractory symptoms and abnormal nonacid reflux by pH impedance monitoring. In their patients, 59% reported symptom improvement postsurgery. They defined preoperative refractory symptoms as <50% improvement following at least 12 weeks of twice-daily PPI therapy. Their patients underwent esophagogastroduodenoscopy, wireless 48-hour pH monitoring, and esophageal motility testing off acid suppression to determine their baseline acid exposure. The patients also underwent 24-hour impedance pH monitoring while on twice-daily PPI therapy. The authors could not confirm that the impedance pH parameter measured while on therapy was a predictor of symptom response following fundoplication.

If endoscopic antireflux therapy is considered, patients should have it only after careful consideration of the alternatives and with clear understanding of the absence of long-term data and the small but real risk for major complications. At present, these procedures should not be considered as indicated for those who have failed medical therapy.

REFERENCES

1. Allison PR. Reflux esophagitis, sliding hiatal hernia, and the anatomy of repair. *Surg Gynecol Obstet.* 1951;92:419–431.

2. Hill LD. An effective operation for hiatal hernia: an eight-year appraisal. *Ann Surg.* 1967;166:681–692.

3. Nissen R. A simple operation to influence reflux esophagitis. *Schweiz Med Wochenschr.* 1956;86(suppl 20):590–592.

4. Geagea T. Laparoscopic Nissen fundoplication: preliminary report on ten cases. *Surg Endosc.* 1991;5:170–173.

5. Bittner HB, Meyers WC, Brazer SR, Pappas TN. Laparoscopic Nissen fundoplication: operative results and short-term follow-up. *Am J Surg.* 1994;167:193–198.

6. Collet D, Cadiere GB. Conversions and complications of laparoscopic treatment of gastroesophageal reflux disease. *Am J Surg.* 1995;169:622–626.

7. Cuschieri A, Hunter J, Wolfe B, et al. Multicenter prospective evaluation of laparoscopic antireflux surgery. *Surg Endosc.* 1993;7:505–510.

8. Fontaumard E, Espalieu P, Boulez J. Laparoscopic Nissen-Rossetti fundoplication. *Surg Endosc.* 1995;9:869–873.

9. Geagea T. Laparoscopic Nissen-Rossetti fundoplication. *Surg Endosc.* 1994;8:1080–1084.

10. Hinder RA, Filipi CJ, Wetscher G, et al. Laparoscopic Nissen fundoplication is an effective treatment for gastroesophageal reflux disease. *Ann Surg.* 1994;220:472–481.

11. Jamieson GG, Watson DI, Britten-Jones R, et al. Laparoscopic Nissen fundoplication. *Ann Surg.* 1994;220:137–145.

12. McKernan JB, Laws HL. Laparoscopic Nissen fundoplication for the treatment of gastroesophageal reflux disease. *Am Surg.* 1994;60: 87–93.

13. McKernan JB, Champion JK. Laparoscopic antireflux surgery. *Am Surg.* 1995;6:530–536.

14. Peters JH, Heimbucher J, Kauer WK, et al. Clinical and physiologic comparison of laparoscopic and open Nissen fundoplication. *J Am Coll Surg.* 1995;180:385–393.

15. Rattner DW, Brooks DC. Patient satisfaction following laparoscopic and open antireflux surgery. *Arch Surg.* 1995;130:289–293.

16. Sataloff DM, Pursnani K, Hoyo S, et al. An objective assessment of laparoscopic antireflux surgery. *Am J Surg.* 1997;174:63–67.

17. Snow LL, Weinstein LS, Hannon JK. Laparoscopic reconstruction of gastroesophageal anatomy for the treatment of reflux disease. *Surg Endosc.* 1995;9:774–780.

18. Weerts JM, Dallemagne B, Hamoir E, et al. Laparoscopic Nissen fundoplication: detailed analysis of 132 patients. *Surg Laparosc Endosc.* 1993;3:359–364.

19. Hetzel DJ, Dent J, Reed WD, et al. Healing and relapse of severe peptic esophagitis after treatment with omeprazole. *Gastroenterology.* 1988;95:903–912.

20. Spechler SJ. Comparison of medical and surgical therapy for complicated gastroesophageal reflux disease in veterans. *N Engl J Med.* 1992;326:786–792.

21. Spechler SJ, Lee E, Ahnen D, et al. Long-term outcome of medical and surgical therapies for gastroesophageal reflux disease. *JAMA.* 2001;285:2331–2338.

22. So JB, Zeitels SM, Rattner DW. Outcomes of atypical symptoms attributed to gastroesophageal reflux treated by laparoscopic fundoplication. *Surgery.* 1998;124:28–32.

23. Johnson WE, Hagen JA, DeMeester TR, et al. Outcome of respiratory symptoms after antireflux surgery on patients with gastroesophageal reflux disease. *Arch Surg.* 1996;131:489–492.

24. DeMeester TR, O'Sullivan GC, Bermudez G, et al. Esophageal function in patients with angina-type chest pain and normal coronary angiograms. *Ann Surg.* 1982;196:488–498.

25. Perrin-Fayolle M, Gormand F, Braillon G, et al. Long-term results of surgical treatment for gastroesophageal reflux in asthmatic patients. *Chest.* 1989;96:40–44.

26. Larrain A, Carrasco E, Galleguillos F, et al. Medical and surgical treatment of nonallergic asthma associated with gastroesophageal reflux. *Chest.* 1991;99:1330–1335.

27. Deveney CW, Benner K, Cohen J. Gastroesophageal reflux and laryngeal disease. *Arch Surg.* 1993;128:1021–1027.

28. Pitcher DE, Pitcher WD, Martin DT, Curet MJ. Antireflux surgery does not reliably correct reflux-related asthma. *Gastrointest Endosc.* 1996;43:433.

29. Hunter JG, Trus TL, Branum GD, et al. A physiological approach to laparoscopic fundoplication for gastroesophageal reflux disease. *Ann Surg.* 1996;223:673–687.

30. Rossetti M, Hell K. Fundoplication for the treatment of gastroesophageal reflux in hiatal hernia. *World J Surg.* 1977;1:439–444.

31. Hunter JG, Pellegrini CA, eds. Surgery of the esophagus. *Surg Clin North Am.* 1977;77:959–1217.

32. Skinner DB, Belsey RHR. *Management of Esophageal Disease.* Philadelphia, PA: WB Saunders; 1988.

33. Hill LD, Kraemer SJM, Aye RW, Kozarek FA, Snopkowski P. Laparoscopic Hill repair. *Contemp Surg*. 1994;1:13–20.

34. Idani H, Asami S, Ishikawa T, et al. Laproscopic tailored Nissen fundoplication. *Surg Endosc*. 2010;24:2221–2225.

35. Kosek V, Wykypiel H, Weiss H, et al. Division of the short gastric vessels during laparoscopic Nissen fundoplication: clinical and functional outcome during long-term follow-up in a prospectively randomized trial. *Surg Endosc*. 2009;23:2208–2213.

36. Schuchert MJ, Pettiford BL, Abbas G, et al. The use of esophageal transit and gastric emptying studies in the evaluation of patients undergoing laparoscopic fundoplication. *Surg Endosc*. 2010;24:3119–3126.

37. Triadafilopoulos G, DiBaise JK, Nostrant TT, et al. The Stretta procedure for the treatment of GERD: 6 and 12 month follow-up of the U.S. open label trial. *Gastrointest Endosc*. 2002;55:149–156.

38. Corley DA, Katz P, Wo JM, et al. Improvement of gastroesophageal reflux symptoms after radiofrequency energy: a randomized, sham-controlled trial. *Gastroenterology*. 2003;125:668–676.

39. Filipi CJ, Lehman GA, Rothstein RI, et al. Transoral, flexible endoscopic suturing for treatment of GERD: a multicenter trial. *Gastrointest Endosc*. 2001;53:416–422.

40. Rothstein RI, Pohl H, Grove M, et al. Endoscopic gastric plication for the treatment of GERD: two-year follow-up results. *Am J Gastroenterol*. 2001;96:S35. Abstract 107.

41. Chen YK, Raijman I, Ben-Menachem T, et al. Long-term outcomes of endoluminal gastroplication: a U.S. multicenter trial. *Gastrointest Endosc*. 2005;61:659–667.

42. Mason RJ, Hughes M, Lehman GA, et al. Endoscopic augmentation of the cardia with a biocompatible injectable polymer (Enteryx) in a porcine model. *Surg Endosc*. 2002;16:386–391.

43. Cohen LB, Johnson DA, Ganz RA, et al. Enteryx implantation for GERD: expanded multicenter trial results and interim postapproval follow-up to 24 months. *Gastrointest Endosc*. 2005;61:650–658.

44. Deviere J, Costamagna G, Neuhaus H, et al. Nonresorbable copolymer implantation for gastroesophageal reflux disease: a randomized sham-controlled multicenter trial. *Gastroenterology*. 2005;128:532–540.

45. Pleskow D, Rothstein R, Lo S, et al. Endoscopic full-thickness plication for the treatment of GERD: 12-month follow-up for the North American open-label trial. *Gastrointest Endosc.* 2005;61:643–649.

46. Pleskow D, Rothstein R, Lo S, et al. Endoscopic full-thickness plication for the treatment of GERD: a multicenter trial. *Gastrointest Endosc.* 2004;59:163–171.

47. Velanovich V. Endoscopic, endoluminal fundoplication for gastroesophageal reflux disease: initial experience and lessons learned. *Surgery.* 2010;148:646–651.

48. Francis DO, Goutte M, Slaughter JC, et al. Traditional reflux parameters and not impedance monitoring predict outcome after fundoplication in extraesophageal reflux. *Laryngoscope.* 2011;121:1902–1909.

Index

Note: Page numbers in **bold** reference nontext material.

A

D

E

I

L

M

N

O

Q

R

T

U